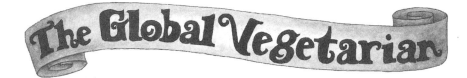

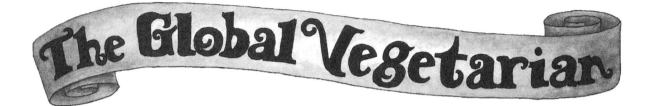

The Global Vegetarian

Adventures in a Meatless Kitchen

Jay Solomon

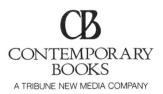

CONTEMPORARY
BOOKS

A TRIBUNE NEW MEDIA COMPANY

Library of Congress Cataloging-in-Publication Data

Solomon, Jay.
    The global vegetarian : adventures in a meatless kitchen / Jay
Solomon.
        p.   cm.
    Includes index.
    ISBN 0-8092-3429-7 (alk. paper)
    1. Vegetarian cookery.   2. Cookery, International   I. Title.
TX837.S682   1995
641.5'636—dc20   95-21542
                                           CIP

Cover illustration by Ronald Wennekes

Published by Contemporary Books, Inc.
Two Prudential Plaza, Chicago, Illinois 60601-6790
Manufactured in the United States of America
International Standard Book Number: 0-8092-3429-7

10   9   8   7   6   5   4   3   2   1

To Emily Page Robin,
my devoted friend and confidant

Other Books by Jay Solomon

Lean Bean Cuisine
A Taste of the Tropics
Global Grilling
Chutneys, Relishes, and Table Sauces

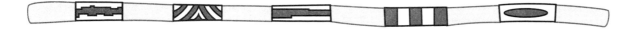

CONTENTS

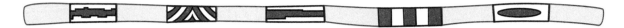

ACKNOWLEDGMENTS

I would like to thank Linda Gray of Contemporary Books for inviting me to write this book. I would also like to thank Carol Martin and Peter Henken of the "Alive and Wellness" nationwide cable show for giving me an opportunity to demonstrate several of these dishes in front of a live television audience. The many students of my Adventures-in-Cooking series at the Green Star Co-Op in Ithaca, New York, have also been a great source of ideas and support.

This is my fifth cookbook, and with each book I have enjoyed the enthusiastic encouragement of friends, family, and relatives. To begin, there are many Solomons to acknowledge: Jesse, Ann, Gregory, Lisa, Heidi, Drew, Margaret, Dick, Margaret Shalaby, and the matriarch of this far-flung extended family, Badia. I prepared many of the dishes for a lively band of taste testers: Emily Robin, Jessica Robin, Beth Ryan, Marilee and Eamonn Murphy, Linda and Jonathan Meyeroff, Leslie Sadoff, Freddi Pollack, Helena Das, Sarah Huber, and Tammy Palmer. In addition, good friends in remote places have continued to express support for my culinary exploits from afar, including Robert and Amy Cima, Shaun Buckley, James Paradiso (and Roseanne), Joe and Vicki Snyder, Riad and Melanie Shalaby, and the whole Robin family. Finally, thanks to Eden Foods for generously donating a variety of beans, grains, soy products, and other staples for my kitchen endeavors.

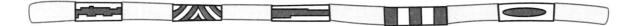

INTRODUCTION

Welcome to the bold new world of *The Global Vegetarian,* a culinary celebration of tantalizing, healthful, and creative recipes. In this book is a bountiful collection of high-spirited, low-fat, meat-free dishes culled from all over the world. The fare is inventive, globally inspired, and at the vanguard of vegetarian cooking.

It's hard to believe that not too long ago vegetarian food was stereotyped as tepid, eccentric, almost antiseptic fare consisting of sprouts, tofu, and granola. To many, a meatless meal was unfathomable. Times have changed, as well as attitudes and tastes. More and more people have discovered the joys of meatless cuisine. In addition, a new generation of imaginative and resourceful cooks have vanquished the outdated notion that meatless meals are unexciting.

As a chef, cooking teacher, and longtime restaurant owner, I have spent many years in the kitchen mincing and slicing, shredding and dicing. I have always approached cooking with a sense of fun, excitement, anticipation, and sometimes even bewilderment. From eloquent feasts to down-home comfort food, a meal is an opportunity to delight the palate, nourish the appetite, and replenish the spirit. It is about thrilling and fulfilling, about creating and indulging.

The Global Vegetarian offers vibrant and worldly recipes for every season and occasion. Each chapter is filled with nourishing and alluring recipes, from morning fare, soups, stews, and appetizers to main entrees, side dishes, and desserts that feature a cornucopia of vegetables and fruits, wholesome grains and pastas, hearty

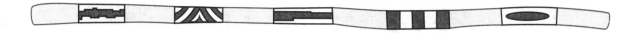

beans and lentils, garden fresh herbs, sprightly chilies, and assertive spices.

In "The Lean Tureen," discover a global melting pot of savory soups, stews, and chilies such as Native Pumpkin and Maize Chowder, Black Bean and Sweet Potato Chili, and Lush Island Squash Bisque. "Worldly Salads" features an entourage of light and rejuvenating salads, including Couscous Tropicale with Black Beans and Corn, Tuscan Bread Salad, and Grilled Tunisian Vegetable Salad.

"Little Bites with Big Flavors" features an eclectic selection of appetizers including Hawaiian Papaya Guacamole, Jamaican Jerk Tempeh, and Sweet Potato Dal. For the main course, "Dinner Mania" portrays world dining at its best: Pumpkin Risotto with Spinach, Creole Eggplant and Black-Eyed Pea Stew, South American Vegetable Stew, Spicy Squash and Chickpea Curry, and West African Jollof Rice are some of the international attractions.

In "Sides That Tantalize," there is a plenitude of supporting side dishes including Lemon-Braised Autumn Greens, Jamaican Cook-Up Rice, Bayou Red Beans and Rice, Stove Top Quinoa Pilaf, and 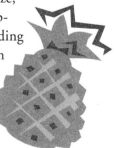 Oven-Roasted Sweet Plantains. When it's time to embellish and adorn, "The Sweet, the Hot, and the Tart" features an array of salsas, chutneys, vinaigrettes, and table sauces including Kiwi Vinaigrette, Mango-Pineapple Chutney, Cucumber Cool Down, and Black Bean Sofrito.

"Arresting Afterthoughts" offers slimmed-down, enlightened versions of sweet quick breads, muffins, and desserts including Zucchini Corn Bread, Sweet Potato–Molasses Muffins, Banana-Rum Rice Pudding, and Chocolate Mocha Tofu Cheesecake. For breakfast and brunch ideas, "Morning Glories" will wake up your taste buds with inspired alternatives to bacon and eggs, featuring Spinach Spuds, Banana Bread French Toast, Pumpkin Buckwheat Pancakes, and Zucchini Crepes with Apple Filling. Finally, "The Guide to the International Pantry" offers an easy-to-use glossary for the well-stocked kitchen.

Here is proof that meatless cuisine need not be uninspiring, boring, or edible only when smothered in cheese. *The Global Vegetarian* taps into the growing parade of seasonal produce, exotic grains, and legumes appearing at the marketplace. Winter squash, root vegetables, and tropical fruits and vegetables abound. Iceberg lettuce is crowded out by cascading leafy green vegetables such as Romaine, escarole, kale, dandelion greens, rapini, frisee, and countless others.

The kitchen cupboard has also expanded. Once there was only white rice; now there are a multitude of grains available, from barley, bulgur, couscous, and brown rice to exotic quinoa, wild rice, and basmati. Yesteryear we all ate spaghetti; today pasta comes in all kinds of shapes, sizes, and colors. There is also a growing variety of beans, peas, and lentils from which to choose.

In *The Global Vegetarian*, you can bid adieu to cream, butter, and other fattening (and unnecessary) ingredients. Instead, a variety of fresh herbs and spices will grace and embrace your palate. Basil, cilantro, thyme, oregano, and mint will accentuate your meal's optimum flavors. The spice cabinet includes ground cumin, curry, turmeric, cayenne pepper, and a wide range of dried herbs. And in this kitchen of heightened flavors, garlic is a cook's best friend, always there to provide comfort.

There are also hot zones throughout the book, opportunities to indulge in a little fire and spice. Peppery hot food, once an ethnic or regional trait, has conquered (and ignited!) America. Instead of reaching for the salt shaker, people are pouring on bottled hot sauce. Jalapeños, poblanos, serranos, and fiery Scotch bonnet chilies have entered our national lexicon of flavors. The piquant sensations these tasty marvels provide further reduces the need for creamy, salty, or buttery flavors.

It is true that health concerns have pushed many people through the doors of meatless dining. Almost every week there is a new announcement about the health benefits of a plant-based diet rich in nutrients and fiber and low in fat, sodium, and cholesterol. The message is clear: a daily diet containing a variety of vegetables, fruits, grains, and legumes offers a reduced risk of coronary heart disease, cancer, and other afflictions. Nutrient-rich foods contribute to a healthful lifestyle and a fuller life. National health organizations, including the National Cancer Institute and The Produce for a Better Health Foundation, ardently campaign for people to eat at least five servings of fruits and vegetables a day along with a high-fiber, low-fat, low-cholesterol diet. The Food Guide Pyramid further articulates the public's need to increase their intake of grains, pastas, vegetables, and fruits, and to use fats and oils sparingly. The signs increasingly point to meatless, cholesterol-free meals.

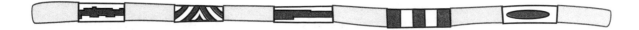

Whether you are a complete vegetarian or merely striving to eat less meat, you will savor the joys of the new meatless cuisine. All you need is a modest affinity for cooking, an appreciation for good, flavorful food, and a taste for adventure. *The Global Vegetarian* is not about slogging through a meal with head bowed down. This is a place to create, innovate, and explore the fertile landscape of the meat-free culinary world.

There has never been a better time to enjoy healthful and adventurous food. Let *The Global Vegetarian* be your gastronomic guide to an enthralling epicurean journey.

Bon appétit, provecho, buon appetito, happy eating!

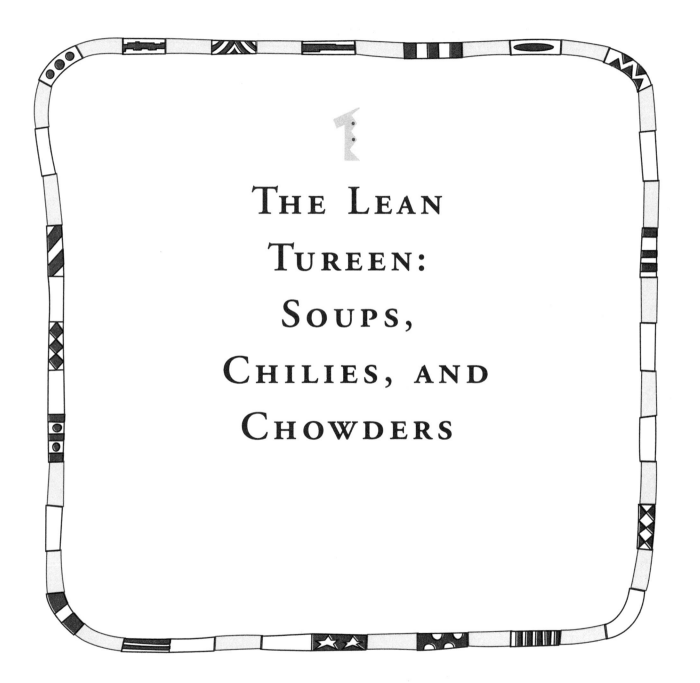

THE LEAN
TUREEN:
SOUPS,
CHILIES, AND
CHOWDERS

Soup, wonderful soup. There is a tureen for every season, a cauldron for every mood. Savory, steaming, bountiful soup simmers on the stove top, beckoning with allure and satisfying nourishment. A well-made soup stimulates the appetite, excites the palate, and soothes the soul. Soup is the ultimate comfort food.

This chapter includes a cornucopia of international and healthful soups, chilies, chowders, gumbos, and bisques. From Portuguese Potato and Kale Soup, Haitian Pumpkin Soup, and Provençal Soupe au Pistou to New World Borscht and Black Bean and Sweet Potato Chili, there is a diverse assortment of one-pot creations. Some are wholly original, while others are improvised versions of classic soup-meals, all prepared without meat, cream, or bouillon cubes, and all high in nutrients, flavor, and substance.

In the meatless kitchen, a harvest of vegetables fills the bowl. Beans, potatoes, root vegetables, and winter squash are natural thickeners, eliminating the need for heavy cream or buttery roux. Thick tomato purees, vegetable stocks, and bean broths lend fluid body while pastas, grains, and legumes add substance. Fresh and dried herbs, garlic, and chili peppers further enhance and romance the broth. With all of these enticing flavors, who needs monotoned canned chicken stocks or salt-laden bouillon cubes? Nobody!

Most soups taste even better the next day, so don't fret about making a large batch. When the soup's on, all is well. The more, the merrier!

HAITIAN PUMPKIN SOUP

While walking along Miami's South Beach, I discovered a Haitian restaurant called Tap Tap. Their pumpkin soup was out of this world (the rum drinks were pretty good, too!), and I couldn't wait to re-create the recipe at home. West Indian pumpkin (called *giraumon* in Haiti), along with potatoes and turnips, are all staples of the Haitian kitchen.

1 tablespoon canola oil
1 medium yellow onion, diced
3 to 4 cloves garlic, minced
1 teaspoon minced Scotch bonnet pepper
  (optional)
5 cups water
4 cups peeled, diced West Indian pumpkin
  or other winter squash such as red kuri,
  butternut, or Hubbard
2 medium turnips, peeled and diced
2 medium carrots, peeled and diced
1 medium unpeeled white potato, chopped
  coarse
8 to 10 whole cloves
2 tablespoons dried parsley
½ teaspoon salt

In a large saucepan, heat the oil. Add the onion, garlic, and, if desired, Scotch bonnet pepper and sauté for about 5 minutes. Add the water, pumpkin, turnips, carrots, potato, and seasonings and cook for 40 to 45 minutes over medium-low heat, stirring occasionally. Let the soup stand for 10 minutes before serving. Ladle into bowls and serve hot.

Makes 8 servings

PORTUGUESE POTATO AND KALE SOUP (CALDO VERDE)

This popular Portuguese soup combines green kale with potatoes (caldo verde means "green soup"). For additional body, I've added white beans instead of the traditional meat. My friend Emily Robin, who lived in Portugal, helped fashion this recipe. "It warmed my stomach on cold rainy days in Lisbon," says Emily.

1 tablespoon olive oil
1 medium yellow onion, chopped
2 to 3 cloves garlic, minced
4 cups water
4 cups diced white potatoes or Yukon Gold potatoes (peeled, if desired)
½ teaspoon white or black pepper
½ teaspoon salt
3 to 4 cups chopped, packed green kale
1 15-ounce can white kidney beans, drained
¼ cup minced parsley

In a large saucepan, heat the oil. Add the onion and garlic and sauté for about 5 minutes. Add the water, potatoes, pepper, and salt and cook for 20 to 25 minutes over medium heat, stirring occasionally.

Stir in the kale, beans, and parsley and cook for 5 to 10 minutes more. To thicken the soup, mash the potatoes against the side of the pan with a wooden spoon. Turn off the heat and let sit for about 10 minutes on the stove top.

Ladle the soup into bowls and serve hot with fresh bread.

Makes 4 to 6 servings

CURRY LENTIL AND SQUASH SOUP

Lentil soup is a popular first course in Middle Eastern and Indian cuisines. When lentils are properly cooked, they should melt in your mouth. This version of the popular soup warms the soul with a flurry of curry.

6 cups water
1 cup green or red lentils, rinsed
½ teaspoon turmeric
1½ tablespoons canola oil
1 large yellow onion, diced
1 cup sliced celery
2 cloves garlic, minced
1 jalapeño pepper or other chili, seeded and
  minced
2 cups peeled, diced butternut or other
  winter squash
2 medium carrots, peeled and diced
1 tablespoon curry powder
1 teaspoon ground cumin
1 teaspoon ground coriander
1 teaspoon salt
½ teaspoon black pepper
¼ teaspoon ground cloves

In a medium saucepan, combine the water, lentils, and turmeric and cook over medium-low heat for about 45 minutes, until the lentils are tender. Set aside.

In a large saucepan, heat the oil. Add the onion, celery, garlic, and jalapeño and sauté for 7 to 10 minutes. Add the squash, carrots, and seasonings and sauté for 1 minute more. Pour in the lentils and cooking liquid and bring to a simmer. Cook over medium heat for 25 to 30 minutes, stirring occasionally.

Serve with a warm flat bread, such as chapati, flour tortilla, pita, or nan.

Makes 6 servings

BEET PASTA FAZOOL

Pasta fazool (slang for "pasta e fagiola") is a nourishing, one-pot meal by itself. This soup is neither dainty nor esoteric, but hearty and copious. Beets help create an enticing scarlet broth brimming with flavor.

1 tablespoon olive oil
1 medium yellow onion, diced
1 small zucchini, diced (about 1 cup)
1 cup sliced celery
8 button mushrooms, sliced (optional)
3 to 4 cloves garlic, minced
3 to 4 medium beets, diced
1 large unpeeled white potato, diced
6 cups water
1 tablespoon dried basil
1 tablespoon dried oregano
1 teaspoon salt
¼ teaspoon red pepper flakes
½ cup uncooked tubetini, ditalini, or other small shell pasta
¼ cup canned tomato paste
1 15-ounce can cannellini beans or Roman beans, drained
2 cups chopped beet greens or escarole (optional)
¼ cup grated Parmesan cheese (optional)

In a large saucepan, heat the oil. Add the onion, zucchini, celery, mushrooms (if desired), and garlic and sauté for 7 minutes. Add the beets, potato, water, and seasonings and simmer for 30 minutes over medium heat, stirring occasionally. Stir in the pasta, tomato paste, beans, and, if desired, greens and simmer for 15 to 20 minutes more, until the pasta is al dente and the beets are tender. Stir occasionally.

Let the soup sit for 10 minutes before serving. Ladle the pasta fazool into bowls and, if desired, sprinkle with the cheese. Serve with warm Italian bread.

Makes 8 servings

KITCHEN TIPS
- If fresh basil or arugula is available, add a handful of the chopped leaves to the soup just before serving.
- When shopping for beets, look for roots with crisp, firm green tops still attached.
- Tubetini and ditalini are tiny pastas available in most grocery stores.

NATIVE PUMPKIN AND MAIZE CHOWDER

Pumpkin and corn (Native Americans called it maize, meaning "life") are indigenous American crops. Pumpkin is loaded with beta-carotene and radiates with a mild, sweet potato–like flavor. Native Americans treated pumpkin like other winter squash and used it for soups, stews, and chowders, often combining it with corn. So there is life for pumpkin beyond holiday pies and Halloween ornaments!

1 tablespoon canola oil
1 medium yellow onion, diced
1 medium green bell pepper, seeded and diced
1 cup sliced celery
2 cloves garlic, minced
6 cups water
4 cups peeled, diced pumpkin, butternut squash, or other winter squash
2 tablespoons dried parsley
1 tablespoon dried thyme leaves
2 teaspoons ground cumin
½ teaspoon salt
½ teaspoon black pepper
2 cups corn kernels, fresh or frozen

In a large saucepan, heat the oil. Add the onion, bell pepper, celery, and garlic and sauté for about 7 minutes. Add the water, pumpkin, and seasonings and cook for 35 to 45 minutes over medium heat, stirring occasionally.

When the pumpkin is tender, stir in the corn and cook for 5 to 10 minutes more. Ladle into bowls and serve hot.

Makes 8 servings

KITCHEN TIPS
- For special occasions, serve the chowder in a baked whole pumpkin (see Index).
- For extra zip, add a minced jalapeño pepper when sautéing the vegetables.
- This soup makes for a great main course when served over rice.

MULLIGATAWNY WITH SQUASH, APPLES, AND TEMPEH

Mulligatawny, which means "pepper water" in Indian parlance, is a robust, brothy soup with an undercurrent of curry. Tempeh, a soybean product rich in protein, adds a "meaty" texture.

> 1 tablespoon canola oil
> 1 large yellow onion, diced
> 1 medium green bell pepper, seeded and diced
> 1 large tomato, diced
> 2 to 3 cloves garlic, minced
> 1 jalapeño or other hot chili pepper, seeded and minced
> 2 to 3 teaspoons curry powder
> 2 teaspoons ground cumin
> ½ teaspoon salt
> ½ teaspoon black pepper
> ¼ teaspoon ground cloves
> 6 cups water
> 2 medium carrots, peeled and diced
> 2 cups peeled, diced butternut squash or sweet potato
> ½ cup long-grain basmati rice (uncooked)
> ¼ cup dark raisins
> 8 ounces tempeh, diced
> 2 medium apples, diced (any variety except Red Delicious)

In a large saucepan, heat the oil. Add the onion, green pepper, tomato, garlic, and jalapeño and sauté for about 7 minutes. Add the seasonings and sauté for 1 minute more. Stir in the water, carrots, squash, rice, and raisins and cook over medium heat for about 10 minutes, stirring occasionally. Stir in the tempeh and apples and cook for 15 to 20 minutes more. Let stand for 10 minutes before serving.

Ladle the mulligatawny into bowls and serve with Indian flat bread (nan or chapati) or pita.

Makes 6 to 8 servings

KITCHEN TIPS

- You can substitute 1 teaspoon of garam masala for the cumin. Or try 1 tablespoon of minced fresh gingerroot in place of the garlic.
- Tempeh is available in the refrigerator section of natural food stores and well-stocked supermarkets. It can also be found in some Asian markets.

POSOLE WITH SWEET POTATOES AND RED BEANS

Posole is a Native American stew of hominy (dried corn kernels), vegetables, beans, and herbs. A cross between a hearty chili and a chunky vegetable stew, posole makes a grand first course for a meatless holiday celebration, especially Thanksgiving or First Night.

1 tablespoon canola oil
1 medium yellow onion, diced
1 medium green bell pepper, seeded and
  diced
1 medium zucchini, diced
2 cloves garlic, minced
4 cups water
1 medium unpeeled sweet or white potato,
  diced
1 15-ounce can hominy, drained and rinsed
1 tablespoon dried oregano
1 tablespoon chili powder
½ teaspoon black pepper
½ teaspoon salt
1 canned chipotle pepper, minced (optional)
1 15-ounce can red kidney beans, drained
2 cups chopped spinach, beet greens, or
  chard
¼ cup canned tomato paste

In a large saucepan, heat the oil. Add the onion, pepper, zucchini, and garlic and sauté for about 7 minutes. Add the water, potato, hominy, seasonings, and, if desired, chipotle pepper. Cook over medium heat for 20 to 25 minutes, stirring occasionally.

Stir in the beans, greens, and tomato paste and cook for 10 to 15 minutes more over low heat. Let stand for 10 minutes before serving.

Makes 8 servings

KITCHEN TIPS

- You can find hominy either canned or frozen in most supermarkets. If using dried hominy, cook the kernels in water for about 3 hours before adding to the recipe.
- For added festivity, serve a sopapilla (a puffy, tortilla-like flat bread) as an accompaniment. Ready-made sopapillas are hard to find outside of the Southwest region, but you can substitute warmed flour tortillas.

WINTRY PARSNIP, SQUASH, AND BEAN STEW

Long ago, before potatoes were commonplace, parsnips were the preferred starch, especially in European kitchens. The off-white, carrot-shaped root vegetable has a mild sweet taste and crunchy texture. It is ideal for soups and stews and pairs up well with two other winter staples, squash and beans.

1 tablespoon canola oil
1 cup sliced celery
2 to 3 cloves garlic, minced
4 large tomatoes, cored and diced
1½ tablespoons sweet paprika
1 tablespoon dried oregano
½ teaspoon salt
2 cups peeled, diced buttercup or butternut squash
2 cups peeled, diced parsnips (about 2 large parsnips)
12 to 16 pearl onions, peeled
1 cup peeled, diced carrots
2½ cups water
1 15-ounce can cranberry beans or red kidney beans, drained
1 cup corn kernels, fresh or frozen
8 broccoli florets

In a large saucepan, heat the oil. Add the celery and garlic and sauté for 3 to 4 minutes. Add the tomatoes and seasonings and cook for about 8 minutes more over medium-low heat, stirring frequently, until the mixture resembles a thick pulp. Add the squash, parsnips, pearl onions, carrots, and water and cook for about 30 minutes, stirring occasionally, until the squash and parsnips are tender. Stir in the beans, corn, and broccoli and cook for 5 to 10 minutes more.

Serve the stew in large serving bowls with brown rice or quinoa on the side.

Makes 4 to 6 servings

KITCHEN TIPS
- Add a minced chipotle pepper for a smoky, peppery nuance.

MISO SOUP WITH UDON

This recipe was inspired by my visits to Japanese noodle shops in New York City. With ease, flamboyance, and animation, line cooks toss, stir, and flip huge cauldrons of noodles, broth, and vegetables. The atmosphere is as appealing as the meal.

Miso, a fermented soybean paste prevalent in Japanese cuisine, brings a delicate flavor to soups. Miso is also nutrient-rich, loaded with protein, and low in fat. Udon, a Japanese noodle made with buckwheat, gives body to the broth, while kombu (dried seaweed) contributes a sealike flavor. Serve the soup with Mesclun Salad Bowl (see Index) or a tossed green salad.

1 tablespoon canola oil
1 medium yellow onion, chopped fine
2 large carrots, peeled and diced
2 cloves garlic, minced
6 cups water or vegetable stock
2 to 3 strips kombu (edible seaweed), soaked in water and diced
4 scallions, chopped
1 2-inch section of daikon, peeled and sliced thin
4 ounces udon (buckwheat noodles), soba, or whole-wheat pasta
2 to 3 tablespoons miso paste
1 cup bean sprouts
Salt and black pepper, to taste

In a large saucepan, heat the oil. Add the onion, carrots, and garlic and sauté over medium heat for about 7 minutes. Add the water or stock, kombu, half of the scallions, and daikon and bring to a simmer. Cook over medium heat for about 5 minutes, then add the udon. (I like to snap the noodles in half before adding to the soup.) Cook over medium-high heat for 12 to 15 minutes, until the noodles are al dente.

Meanwhile, dissolve the miso paste in 2 to 3 tablespoons warm water. Just before serving, stir the miso paste into the soup. Do not boil the soup once the miso paste has been added.

Ladle the soup into large bowls and top with the bean sprouts and the remaining scallions. Season with salt and pepper at the table.

Makes 6 servings

KITCHEN TIPS

- If you have the time and resources, you can add dashi in place of the water. Dashi is a stock made by simmering water and kombu (dried seaweed) for 20 to 30 minutes. The resulting liquid forms the basis of most Japanese soups and sauces.
- Miso paste can be found in many Asian markets and near the soy sauce in well-stocked grocery stores.
- Look for kombu, daikon, and udon in Asian grocery stores and well-stocked markets.

TOMATO-VEGETABLE AND GNOCCHI SOUP

This is a wholesome mélange of vegetables, herbs, and gnocchi (a pasta dumpling made with potatoes). For a light meal, serve the soup with Italian bread and Emily's Spinach and Shredded Beet Salad (see Index).

 1½ tablespoons canola oil
 1 medium yellow onion, diced
 1 cup sliced celery
 1 medium green bell pepper, seeded and
   diced
 1 small zucchini, diced
 6 to 8 medium button mushrooms, sliced
 2 medium-size ripe tomatoes, diced
 1 28-ounce can crushed tomatoes
 4 cups water
 2 tablespoons fresh minced parsley
   (or 1 tablespoon dried)
 1 tablespoon dried basil
 1 tablespoon dried oregano
 1 teaspoon black pepper
 ½ teaspoon salt
 ½ pound gnocchi, fresh or frozen

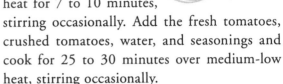

In a large saucepan, heat the oil. Add all of the vegetables except the tomatoes and cook over medium heat for 7 to 10 minutes, stirring occasionally. Add the fresh tomatoes, crushed tomatoes, water, and seasonings and cook for 25 to 30 minutes over medium-low heat, stirring occasionally.

Stir in the gnocchi. Cook according to package directions, until the gnocchi is tender.

Ladle the soup into bowls and serve hot.

Makes 6 to 8 servings

KITCHEN TIPS
- Try sprinkling grated Parmesan or shredded mozzarella cheese over the soup before serving.
- For more greenery, stir in shredded kale or rapini along with the gnocchi. Corn kernels or green peas may also be added.

RISOTTO SOUP WITH SPINACH AND BUTTERNUT SQUASH

Risotto, an Italian rice dish, is transformed into a delightful creamy soup here. The key is to use arborio rice, an Italian grain that cooks up creamy, not fluffy like other rices. The squash, spinach, and rice meld together to form an eloquent unison. *Delizioso.*

1½ tablespoons canola oil
1 medium yellow onion, chopped fine
1 medium red bell pepper, seeded and diced
2 to 3 cloves garlic, minced
5 cups water
4 cups peeled, chopped butternut squash
¾ cup arborio rice
½ teaspoon salt
½ teaspoon white pepper
1 cup chopped frozen spinach (or 2 cups fresh)
½ cup grated Parmesan cheese

In a large saucepan, heat the oil. Add the onion, bell pepper, and garlic and sauté for 5 to 7 minutes. Add the water, squash, rice, and seasonings and cook over medium heat for 20 minutes, stirring occasionally. Stir in the spinach and cook for about 10 minutes more over low heat.

Remove from the heat and stir in the Parmesan cheese. Ladle the soup into bowls and serve hot, with extra Parmesan cheese at the table.

Makes 8 servings

LUSH ISLAND SQUASH BISQUE

This bisque dances on the taste buds with much animation and liveliness. It flickers with heat, gingerroot, and curry. I tasted a version of this soup while on a culinary excursion to St. Lucia, an intoxicatingly beautiful island in the Caribbean.

1 tablespoon canola oil
1 large yellow onion, diced
1 cup sliced celery
4 cloves garlic, minced
1 tablespoon minced gingerroot
1 jalapeño or other hot chili, seeded and
*   minced (optional)*
2 large tomatoes, diced
1 tablespoon curry powder
2 teaspoons ground cumin
1 teaspoon ground coriander
1 teaspoon salt
½ teaspoon black pepper
¼ teaspoon ground cloves
4 cups peeled, diced West Indian pumpkin,
*   butternut squash, or other winter squash*
5 cups water

In a large saucepan, heat the oil. Add the onion, celery, garlic, gingerroot, and, if desired, chili and sauté for about 5 minutes. Add the tomatoes and sauté for 3 to 4 minutes more. Stir in the seasonings and cook for 1 minute more, stirring frequently. Add the squash and water and cook for 30 to 35 minutes over medium heat, stirring occasionally.

Cool for about 10 minutes and then transfer to a food processor fitted with a steel blade (or to a blender) and process for about 15 seconds, until smooth. Return the bisque to the pan and bring to a simmer. Ladle into bowls and serve hot.

Makes 6 servings

PROVENÇAL SOUPE AU PISTOU

This aromatic dish is the French version of minestrone. (The French may say that minestrone is the Italian version of soupe au pistou.) The soup is cooked stew-style, in one large pot, and the pistou, a rich paste of basil, garlic, and cheese, is swirled in at the table. Pistou sounds a little like "pesto," and the ingredients are indeed similar.

FOR THE SOUP:

1 tablespoon canola oil

1 medium yellow onion, diced

1 cup diced celery

2 cups chopped leeks, well rinsed

6 cups water

2 cups diced white potatoes (peeled if desired)

2 tablespoons dried parsley

1 tablespoon dried basil

1 teaspoon white pepper

1 teaspoon salt

1½ cups green string beans, cut into 1-inch sections

1 15-ounce can cannellini or Navy beans, drained

1 cup pasta spirals or ½ cup ditalini or tubetini

FOR THE PISTOU:

6 to 8 cloves garlic, minced

1 cup chopped basil leaves

⅓ cup olive oil

¼ to ½ cup grated Parmesan cheese

In a large saucepan, heat the oil. Add the onion, celery, and leeks and sauté for about 7 minutes, until tender. Add the water, potatoes, and seasonings and bring to a simmer over medium-low heat. Cook for 20 to 25 minutes. Add the green beans, cannellini or Navy beans, and pasta and cook for about 15 minutes more over low heat, stirring occasionally.

Meanwhile, make the pistou: crush the garlic and basil together in a bowl or blender. Blend in the oil and cheese, forming a paste. Transfer to a serving bowl.

Ladle the soup into bowls. Spoon about 1 tablespoon of pistou over the top of each bowl of soup. Pass the remaining pistou at the table.

Makes 8 servings

KITCHEN TIPS

- In post-basil autumn, try using arugula instead.
- Soupe au pistou's ingredients change with the seasons (depending on what's available) so there is no single recipe. When the time is right, try adding parsnips, carrots, zucchini, or winter squash.

NEW WORLD BORSCHT

Borscht, an old-world classic, is reinvigorated in a new-world kitchen. Parsnips and apples add a subtle sweetness, and the result is as pleasing to the eye as it is to the palate. This soup can be served hot or cold (I prefer it hot).

1 tablespoon canola oil
1 medium yellow onion, diced
1 cup sliced celery
2 cloves garlic, minced
4 cups water
2 cups peeled, diced beets (3 to 4 beets)
2 cups peeled, diced parsnips (about 2 parsnips)
2 tablespoons minced parsley
½ teaspoon dried thyme
½ teaspoon nutmeg
½ teaspoon black pepper
½ teaspoon salt
1 large apple (any variety except Red Delicious), cored and diced

In a large saucepan, heat the oil. Add the onion, celery, and garlic and cook for about 7 minutes over medium heat, stirring frequently. Add the water, beets, parsnips, and seasonings and cook for 40 minutes, stirring occasionally. Stir in the apple and cook for 10 to 15 minutes more, until the beets and parsnips are tender.

Transfer the mixture to a food processor fitted with a steel blade (or to a blender) and puree until smooth. Serve immediately, or refrigerate for 2 to 4 hours before serving.

If you'd like, top with light sour cream, low-fat yogurt, or Cucumber Cool Down (see Index).

Makes 6 servings

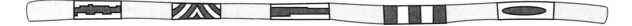

RUSTIC POTATO AND BROCCOLI BISQUE

Bisques connotate a creamy soup, and some bisques call for more cream than you'll find in ice cream. This lighter version calls for low-fat milk and potatoes, and has significantly less fat and calories. The broccoli stalks, chopped up like celery, add additional substance.

2 bunches fresh broccoli (about 2 pounds)
1 tablespoon canola oil
2 small yellow onions, diced
1 cup sliced celery
2 to 3 cloves garlic, minced
5 cups water
4 cups unpeeled, diced white potatoes
½ cup dry sherry
*¼ cup chopped fresh parsley (or 2
 tablespoons dried)*
1 teaspoon nutmeg
1 teaspoon dried thyme leaves
¾ teaspoon salt
½ teaspoon black pepper
¼ teaspoon white pepper
2 cups low-fat milk

Chop the broccoli florets from the stalks. Finely chop 1 to 2 of the broccoli stalks (enough to fill 1 cup).

In a large saucepan, heat the oil. Add the onion, celery, garlic, and chopped broccoli stalks and sauté over medium heat for 7 to 10 minutes. Add the water, potatoes, sherry, and seasonings and bring to a simmer. Cook for about 25 minutes over medium heat, stirring occasionally. Reduce the heat to low, stir in the broccoli florets and milk, and cook for 10 minutes more.

Transfer one-fourth of the soup to a food processor fitted with a steel blade (or to a blender) and process for 10 to 15 seconds. Pour into a mixing bowl and repeat, until all of the soup has been processed. Return the soup to the pan and keep warm until ready to serve.

Ladle into bowls and serve hot.

Makes 8 to 10 servings

HARVEST CORN CHOWDER

I live for harvest time. Farmers' markets overflow with the local bounty, my garden comes to fruition, and there is a festive mood in the air. This chowder epitomizes the spirit of the harvest. Winter squash melds into the simmering liquid and forms a thick, delicious stock, eliminating the need for cream or a butter-based roux, while parsnips and corn add body.

1 tablespoon canola oil
2 cups chopped leeks, well rinsed
1 cup sliced celery
1 medium red bell pepper, seeded and diced
2 to 3 cloves garlic, minced
4½ cups water
2 cups peeled, diced parsnips or white
    potatoes
2 cups peeled, diced buttercup, butternut,
    sugar pie pumpkin, or other winter squash
2 cups corn kernels, fresh or frozen
¼ cup dry sherry
2 tablespoons dried parsley
1 tablespoon dried oregano
2 teaspoons paprika
1 teaspoon dried thyme leaves
½ teaspoon salt
½ teaspoon black pepper

In a large saucepan, heat the oil. Add the leeks, celery, pepper, and garlic and sauté for 7 minutes, until the vegetables are tender. Add the remaining ingredients (except the corn, if frozen) and bring to a simmer. Cook over medium heat for about 35 to 40 minutes, stirring occasionally, until the parsnips are tender and the squash has liquified. (Add the corn if it is frozen and return to a gentle simmer for about 5 minutes.)

Ladle into bowls and serve with a hearth-style bread.

Makes 4 to 6 servings

BLACK BEAN AND SWEET POTATO CHILI

Chili has come a long way from its former meat-laden sloppy Joe-look-alike days. This hearty recipe offers a smoldering cauldron of earthy black beans, vegetables, and assertive spices.

1 tablespoon canola oil
1 medium yellow onion, diced
1 medium green bell pepper, seeded and diced
1 cup sliced celery
2 cloves garlic, minced
1 jalapeño pepper, seeded and minced
2 tomatoes, cored and diced
2 15-ounce cans black beans, drained
1 28-ounce can crushed tomatoes
1 tablespoon chili powder
1 tablespoon dried parsley (or 2 tablespoons fresh)
2 teaspoons ground cumin
½ teaspoon black pepper
½ teaspoon salt
2 cups unpeeled, diced sweet potato (about 1 large potato)
1 red onion or 4 scallions, chopped (optional)

In a large saucepan, heat the oil. Add the onion, bell pepper, celery, garlic, and jalapeño and cook for 7 minutes over medium heat, stirring frequently. Stir in the tomatoes and cook for 3 to 4 minutes more. Stir in the beans, crushed tomatoes, and seasonings and cook for about 30 minutes over medium-low heat, stirring occasionally.

In a medium saucepan, place the sweet potatoes in enough boiling water to cover. Cook for about 15 minutes over medium heat, until tender, and drain in a colander. When the chili has cooked for about 25 minutes, stir the potatoes into the pot.

Ladle the chili into bowls and garnish with chopped red onion or scallions. Serve with Zucchini Corn Bread and Cucumber Cool Down (see Index for recipes).

Makes 6 servings

SUN-DRIED TOMATO CHILI

If you can't bear the sight or taste of a rubbery tomato in midwinter, sun-dried tomatoes make an attractive alternative. They bring a rustic essence to this vegetable chili. If given the choice, choose air-packed dried tomatoes over the oil-drenched variety.

1 cup sun-dried tomatoes
1½ tablespoons canola oil
1 large yellow onion, diced
1 medium green bell pepper, seeded and
* diced*
1 cup sliced celery
1 28-ounce can crushed tomatoes
1 15-ounce can red kidney beans, drained
1 tablespoon chili powder
1 tablespoon dried oregano
1½ teaspoons ground cumin
1 to 2 teaspoons Tabasco or other bottled
* hot sauce*
½ teaspoon salt
½ teaspoon black pepper
1 to 2 cups chopped spinach, mizuna, or
* other winter leafy green*

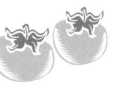

Soak the tomatoes in hot water for about 30 minutes. Drain and coarsely chop.

In a large saucepan, heat the oil. Add the onion, bell pepper, and celery and sauté for 6 to 8 minutes, until the vegetables are tender. Stir in the tomatoes, canned tomatoes, beans, and seasonings and simmer for about 20 minutes over medium-low heat, stirring occasionally. Stir in the spinach and cook for 10 minutes more.

Ladle the chili into bowls and serve hot.

Makes 4 to 6 servings

KITCHEN TIPS
- Serve with a variety of garnishes such as shredded low-fat provolone cheese, diced red onion, chopped scallions, and fresh cilantro or basil.
- Mizuna is a tasty Japanese winter green that is available in natural food stores and well-stocked supermarkets.

WHITE BEAN, CORN, AND EGGPLANT CHILI

Once the idea of making a meatless chili takes root, a whole range of culinary possibilities comes to light. This Southwestern-inspired chili is a prime example of the alluring alternatives to humdrum meat chili.

1½ tablespoons canola oil
1 large yellow onion, diced
1 medium red or green bell pepper, seeded and diced
2 cups unpeeled, diced eggplant
2 cloves garlic, minced
2 cups corn kernels, fresh or frozen
1 15-ounce can white kidney beans, drained
1 15-ounce can stewed tomatoes
2 tablespoons dried parsley
1 tablespoon dried oregano
½ teaspoon salt
½ teaspoon black pepper
2 to 3 ounces shredded part-skim mozzarella, low-fat provolone, or Swiss cheese

In a large saucepan, heat the oil. Add the onion, bell pepper, eggplant, and garlic and cook over medium heat for about 10 minutes, stirring occasionally, until the vegetables are tender. Stir in the corn, beans, tomatoes, and seasonings. Cook for about 20 minutes over low heat, stirring frequently.

Ladle into bowls and swirl the cheese into the chili.

Makes 4 to 6 servings

KITCHEN TIPS
- You may also top the chili with chopped watercress, arugula, or cilantro.

RED BEAN AND QUINOA CHILI

Quinoa (pronounced keen-wa) is an ancient grain native to the highlands of South America. Here it unites with down-to-earth red beans for a nourishing chili that is full of nutrients and flavor. It is a perfect dish to eat before (or after) a day of high-energy activities.

1 cup quinoa, rinsed
2 cups water
1 tablespoon canola oil
1 large yellow onion, diced
1 medium green bell pepper, seeded and diced
1 cup sliced celery
1 large carrot, peeled and diced
1 jalapeño pepper, seeded and minced
2 tomatoes, cored and diced
2 15-ounce cans red kidney beans or black beans, drained
1 28-ounce can crushed tomatoes
1 tablespoon chili powder
1 tablespoon dried parsley (or 2 tablespoons fresh)
1 tablespoon dried oregano
2 teaspoons ground cumin
½ teaspoon black pepper
½ teaspoon salt
4 scallions, chopped (optional)

In a medium saucepan, combine the quinoa and water and cover. Bring to a simmer over medium heat and cook for 15 to 20 minutes, until all of the liquid is absorbed. Remove from the heat and let stand for about 10 minutes.

In a large saucepan, heat the oil. Add the onion, bell pepper, celery, carrot, and jalapeño and cook for 7 minutes over medium heat, stirring frequently. Stir in the tomatoes and cook for 3 to 4 minutes more. Stir in the beans, crushed tomatoes, and seasonings and cook for about 25 minutes over low heat, stirring occasionally. Stir in the quinoa and cook for 5 minutes more.

Ladle the chili into bowls. Top with scallions, if desired, and serve.

Makes 8 servings

RIBOLLITA

Ribollita means "reboiled" in Italian. The idea—reheating yesterday's soup and pouring it over stale bread—sounds unremarkable, but the result is truly satisfying. This minestrone-style soup, sated with white beans, vegetables, and herbs, has a humble peasant origin but radiates with sophisticated flavor.

2 tablespoons olive oil
1 medium yellow onion, diced
2 cloves garlic, minced
1 small zucchini or eggplant, diced
1 cup shredded red or white cabbage
2 medium carrots, peeled and diced
6 cups water
1 28-ounce can whole tomatoes, undrained
2 cups unpeeled, diced white potatoes
1 tablespoon dried basil
1 teaspoon sage
½ teaspoon salt
½ teaspoon red pepper flakes
½ pound fresh green beans, cut into 1-inch
  lengths (about 2 cups)
1 small (about 12-ounce) loaf Italian bread,
  torn into bite-size pieces

In a large saucepan, heat the oil. Add the onion and garlic and sauté for about 5 minutes, until translucent. Add the zucchini, cabbage, and carrots and cook over medium heat for about 10 minutes, stirring frequently. Stir in the water, undrained tomatoes, potatoes, and seasonings and bring to a simmer. Cook for about 45 minutes over medium heat, stirring occasionally. Stir in the green beans and simmer for about 5 minutes more.

Remove from the heat and let cool for several minutes. Serve immediately or cover and chill for later.

When ready to eat, reheat the soup (if necessary) in a large saucepan over low heat, until it simmers. Place the torn bread into the bottom of each soup bowl. Ladle the soup over the bread and pack it down with a spoon. Let the soup sit for a few minutes, allowing the bread to soak in the broth.

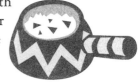

Makes 8 servings

GUMBO Z'HERBES
WITH BEAN BROTH

Gumbo came to the Americas from Africa, where it literally means okra. Although most gumbos contain meat, Gumbo Z'Herbes (also known as green gumbo) is a meatless version served during the Lenten season. Legend has it that for every variety of greens placed in the gumbo, a new friend would be made—so, although I only call for spinach, feel free to add a mixture of beet greens, mustard greens, dandelions, kale, or carrot tops as well.

½ cup red kidney beans, soaked overnight and drained
8 cups water
1½ tablespoons canola oil
1 medium yellow onion, diced
1 medium green or red bell pepper, seeded and diced
1 cup sliced celery
2 cloves garlic, minced
1 16-ounce can crushed tomatoes
2 medium carrots, peeled and diced
2 tablespoons dried parsley
1 tablespoon dried oregano
1 teaspoon dried thyme
½ teaspoon black pepper
¼ teaspoon cayenne pepper
½ teaspoon salt
1 cup frozen chopped okra
1½ cups frozen chopped spinach (or 3 cups fresh)
4 cups cooked white or brown rice
2 scallions, chopped

In a large saucepan, combine the beans and water and cook over medium heat for 1 to 1½ hours, until the beans are tender. Drain, reserving 4 cups of the broth.

In a large saucepan, heat the oil. Add the onion, bell pepper, celery, and garlic and sauté for about 7 minutes, until the vegetables are tender. Add the beans, broth, crushed tomatoes, carrots, and seasonings and cook over medium-low heat for 15 minutes, stirring occasionally. Stir in the okra and spinach and cook for about 15 minutes more.

Place ½ cup cooked rice in the bottom of each soup bowl. Ladle the gumbo over the rice and top with scallions. Serve with Chili Corn Bread (see Index).

Makes 8 servings

KITCHEN TIPS
- You can use the same amount of fresh okra in place of the frozen. When using fresh okra, add it to the soup along with the beans, broth, and other ingredients.

CARROT VICHYSSOISE

Vichyssoise, the classic potato and leek soup of French pedigree, is jazzed up here with beta-carotene–rich carrots. This versatile soup can be enjoyed hot in the winter or cold during the summer.

1 tablespoon canola oil
1 medium yellow onion, diced
2 cups chopped leeks (about 1 large leek)
2 cups peeled, diced carrots
4 cups water
2 cups peeled, coarsely chopped white
  potatoes
2 tablespoons dried parsley
1 teaspoon salt
1 teaspoon white pepper
2 cups low-fat milk
¼ cup chopped chives

In a large saucepan, heat the oil. Add the onion, leeks, and carrots and sauté over medium heat for 7 to 10 minutes, until the vegetables are tender. Add the water, potatoes, and dried seasonings and bring to a simmer. Cook over medium-low heat for about 35 minutes, stirring occasionally. Add the milk and return to a simmer. Remove the soup from the heat and let cool for a few minutes.

Transfer the soup to a blender or food processor fitted with a steel blade and puree until smooth. Ladle into bowls and serve hot, or chill for later. Sprinkle chives over the soup before serving.

Makes 8 servings

CRIOLLA STEW WITH SPICY CORN DUMPLINGS

Creole cooking in the Caribbean is known as "comida criolla." It is a melting pot of French, Spanish, African, and native island cuisines.

FOR THE CORN DUMPLINGS:

> ½ cup fine cornmeal
> ½ cup unbleached all-purpose flour
> ½ teaspoon baking powder
> ½ teaspoon salt
> 1 jalapeño pepper, seeded and minced
> 5 to 6 tablespoons water

FOR THE STEW:

> 1 tablespoon canola oil
> 1 medium yellow onion, diced
> 1 medium green bell pepper, seeded and diced
> 1 chayote squash or small zucchini, peeled and diced
> 2 to 3 cloves garlic, minced
> 6 cups water or vegetable stock
> 2 cups peeled, diced butternut squash, sweet potato, or West Indian pumpkin
> 2 tablespoons dried parsley
> 2 teaspoons dried thyme leaves
> ½ teaspoon black pepper
> ½ teaspoon salt
> ½ teaspoon allspice
> 1 whole Scotch bonnet pepper (optional)

Make the dumplings: In a mixing bowl, combine the cornmeal, flour, baking powder, salt, and jalapeño. Gradually add the water, forming a moist, pliable dough. Divide the dough into 8 equal balls. Set aside.

Make the stew: In a large saucepan, heat the oil. Add the onion, bell pepper, squash, and garlic and sauté for about 7 minutes. Add the water, butternut squash, and seasonings and bring to a simmer. If desired (and if you are brave), puncture the Scotch bonnet pepper with a fork and add, whole, to the stew. Add the dumplings and cook for 30 to 35 minutes over medium heat, stirring occasionally.

Remove the Scotch bonnet pepper from the stew. Discard or seed, cut into strips, and give it to a hot foods aficionado. Ladle the stew into bowls, making sure everyone gets a dumpling.

Makes 8 servings

KITCHEN TIPS

- Chayote squash is a pear-shaped, pale green Caribbean squash with a firm texture and mild flavor. It is available in Hispanic and Caribbean markets and in the specialty produce section of well-stocked grocery stores.

ROOT VEGETABLE VICHYSSOISE

Although the root vegetable family is a humble lot, when given the chance, turnips, rutabagas, and parsnips can inspire delicious soups and stews. This recipe is delicious proof.

1½ tablespoons canola oil
1 medium yellow onion, diced
2 cups chopped leeks (about 1 large leek)
5 cups water
2 cups peeled, diced white potatoes or parsnips
1 cup peeled, diced rutabagas
1 cup peeled, diced turnips
3 to 4 tablespoons dried parsley
1 teaspoon salt
1 teaspoon white pepper
2 cups low-fat milk
¼ cup chopped scallions
¼ to ½ cup shredded Gouda or Gruyère cheese (optional)

In a large saucepan, heat the oil. Add the onion and leeks and sauté over medium heat for 7 to 10 minutes, until tender. Add the water, potatoes, rutabagas, turnips, and dried seasonings and bring to a simmer. Cook over medium-low heat for about 45 minutes to 1 hour, stirring occasionally. Add the milk and return to a simmer. Remove the soup from the heat and let cool for a few minutes.

Transfer the soup to a blender or food processor fitted with a steel blade and puree until smooth. Ladle into bowls and serve hot, or chill for later and serve as a cold soup. Before serving, top with a sprinkle of scallions and, if desired, a smidgeon of shredded Gouda or Gruyère cheese.

Makes 8 servings

CALYPSO PEPPERPOT WITH TROPICAL TUBERS

Pepperpot is a Caribbean soup made with a variety of ingredients including pumpkin, yams, yuca, and whatever else is in the kitchen. Callaloo, a leafy green vegetable similar to spinach, is another main ingredient (although spinach or Swiss chard may be substituted).

1½ tablespoons canola oil
1 large yellow onion, diced
1 medium green bell pepper, seeded and diced
½ Scotch bonnet pepper or other hot chili, seeded and minced
3 to 4 cloves garlic, minced
5 cups water
1 plantain, peeled and chopped coarse
1 cup peeled, diced Caribbean yams, dasheen, or sweet potatoes
1 cup peeled, diced yuca
2 tablespoons dried parsley
2 teaspoons dried thyme leaves
½ teaspoon black pepper
½ teaspoon allspice
1 teaspoon salt
2 to 3 cups chopped callaloo, spinach, or Swiss chard
4 scallions, chopped
1 to 1½ cups reduced-fat coconut milk

In a large saucepan, heat the oil. Add the onion, bell pepper, chili, and garlic and sauté for about 7 minutes. Add the water, plantain, yams, yuca, and seasonings and cook over medium heat for about 45 minutes to 1 hour, until the tubers are tender, stirring occasionally. Stir in the callaloo, scallions, and coconut milk and cook for 15 minutes more over low heat. Let stand for 10 minutes before serving.

Ladle into bowls and serve hot.

Makes 8 servings

KITCHEN TIPS
- Callaloo, along with plantains, yuca, and many other tropical tubers can be found in Caribbean and Hispanic markets as well as the specialty produce sections of well-stocked grocery stores.

GREG'S GARDEN GAZPACHO

Gazpacho is Spain's gift to the world. This is my brother Greg's gift to my cookbook. He adds bulgur and a plethora of garden vegetables to this delightful dish. It is a refreshing antidote for a hot, humid day.

¼ cup fine bulgur (cracked wheat)
1 cup hot water
2 large ripe tomatoes, diced
1 small yellow onion, diced
1 small green or red bell pepper, seeded and diced
1 small cucumber, peeled and diced
1 small jalapeño or serrano pepper, seeded and minced
2 cloves garlic, minced
½ cup chopped parsley
2 to 4 tablespoons chopped basil
1 teaspoon Tabasco or other bottled hot sauce
¼ teaspoon black pepper
¼ teaspoon salt
2 cups tomato juice or V-8 juice
4 sprigs fresh basil or mint

Soak the bulgur in the hot water for about 30 minutes. Drain and discard any excess liquid.

Place all of the remaining ingredients (except the fresh basil or mint sprigs) in a blender or food processor fitted with a steel blade. Process for 5 to 10 seconds, forming a vegetable mash. Transfer to a large bowl and blend in the bulgur. Chill for at least 1 hour before serving. Serve in chilled bowls and garnish with sprigs of fresh basil or mint.

Makes 4 servings

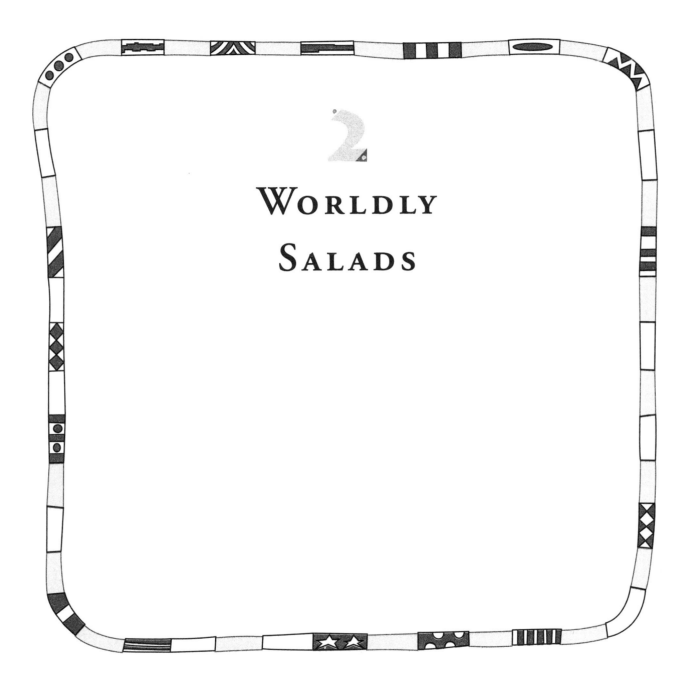

2

WORLDLY
SALADS

well-made salad can be a wonderful thing. Depending on your mood and appetite, a salad can serve as a stimulating first course, a light entree, or a cleanser for an already sated palate. It may be a bowl of leafy greens dressed with a vinaigrette. Or a plate of cold pasta and beans tossed lightly with an herb marinade. It could be couscous, corn, and scallions simply sprayed with a mist of lime. Today's salads are diverse and versatile.

Not too long ago a tossed salad meant a bowl of lifeless iceberg lettuce submerged in a river of gooey, lavalike dressing. Potato salads often involved a mudslide of heavy mayonnaise. Thankfully, whether it was due to a rebellion or natural progression, the world of salads has changed. Now, more than ever, rejuvenated salads play a significant role in the healthful regime.

In this chapter there are a plethora of enticing salad combinations ranging from Cuban Black Bean and Rice Salad and Pear, Arugula, and Chard Salad to the classic Tuscan Bread Salad, an exotic Peppery Quinoa and Mixed Bean Salad, and a refreshing Mesclun Salad Bowl. This is a compendium of light and healthful salads prepared with a variety of greens, vegetables, grains, and pastas.

The big news in salads is the burgeoning selection of leafy green vegetables that are available. Dowdy iceberg pales in comparison to sturdy Romaine, red and green leaf, Swiss chard, escarole, curly endive, dandelion greens, rapini, frisee, and mizuna. Leafy greens bring a host of valuable nutrients and fresh flavors to the salad arena. (As a rule, the darker the leaf, the more vitamins and minerals are present.)

Of course, salads are not limited to tossed greens. In the meatless *garde mangier*, there are beets, carrots, parsnips, green beans, summer squash, jicama, apples, and many other vegetables and fruits. In addition, stellar combinations of grains, beans, and pastas transform a salad into a satisfying light entree. Many of the contemporary dressings are derived from vinegar, citrus juice, low-fat yogurt, and herbs, offering less calories and fat—and more flavor—than the heavy concoctions of the past. Mustard, horseradish, garlic, and chilies provide additional depth and diversity.

BLACK-EYED PEA, CORN, AND SWEET POTATO SALAD

This is an example of how simple, ordinary ingredients—legumes, corn, potatoes—can combine to form extraordinary flavors. You can enjoy this salad year-round, but it's especially appropriate around New Year's Day, when eating black-eyed peas is thought to bring good luck for the coming year.

2 cups unpeeled, diced sweet potatoes
2 tablespoons canola oil
2 tablespoons red wine vinegar
1 teaspoon Dijon-style mustard
¼ cup chopped fresh parsley (or 2 tablespoons dried)
½ teaspoon black pepper
¼ teaspoon salt
2 15-ounce cans black-eyed peas, drained
1½ cups corn kernels, fresh or frozen and thawed
2 scallions, chopped fine
6 to 8 large pieces leaf lettuce (optional)

In a medium saucepan, place the sweet potatoes in enough boiling water to cover and cook for about 15 minutes over medium heat, until tender. Drain and cool under cold running water.

Meanwhile, in a large mixing bowl, whisk together the oil, vinegar, mustard, and seasonings. Blend in the black-eyed peas, corn, scallions, and sweet potatoes. Chill for at least 1 hour before serving. Place over a bed of leaf lettuce.

Makes 6 servings

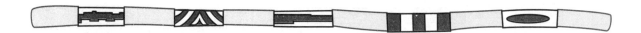

NEW AMERICAN POTATO SALAD WITH BEETS AND APPLES

The American potato salad has been long overdue for a makeover. In the past, the salad has too often been a gummy mass collapsed beneath the weight of too much mayonnaise. For a new approach to this old standard, try a light mustard vinaigrette and two colorful additions, beets and apples.

2 cups scrubbed, diced fresh beets
2 cups unpeeled, diced white or red potatoes
3 to 4 tablespoons canola oil
2 tablespoons apple cider vinegar
2 teaspoons Dijon-style mustard
2 tablespoons chopped parsley
½ teaspoon black pepper
½ teaspoon salt
½ cup minced red onion
1 cup diced celery
2 red apples, unpeeled and diced

In a medium saucepan, place the beets in enough boiling water to cover and cook for 20 to 25 minutes, until the beets are easily pierced with a fork, but are still firm. Drain and cool under cold running water. (Or wrap 3 to 4 whole beets in aluminum foil and bake at 375°F for 50 minutes to 1 hour, until tender. Cool and dice the beets.)

In a medium saucepan, place the potatoes in enough boiling water to cover and cook for about 15 minutes, until easily pierced with a fork. Drain and cool under cold running water.

Meanwhile, in a large mixing bowl, whisk together the oil, vinegar, mustard, parsley, and seasonings. Blend in the red onion, celery, and apples. When the beets and potatoes are ready, toss with the vinaigrette mixture. Chill for 1 hour before serving.

Makes 6 servings

KITCHEN TIPS
- If fresh herbs are in season, add a few tablespoons of chopped dill, tarragon, or basil.

RATSIE'S PASTA SALAD WITH HERB-PARMESAN VINAIGRETTE

When restaurateur and friend Jim Paradiso asked me to invent a new salad for his popular eatery in College Park, Maryland, I came up with this summertime creation. The key flavors are provided by a combination of fresh and dried herbs and balsamic vinegar, a well-aged wine vinegar with a smooth aftertaste.

½ pound pasta spirals (fusilli) or rotini
3 tablespoons olive oil
2 tablespoons balsamic vinegar or red wine
*   vinegar*
1 tablespoon Dijon-style mustard
2 cloves garlic, minced
3 tablespoons chopped parsley
3 tablespoons chopped basil
2 tablespoons chopped oregano
1 tablespoon dried oregano
½ teaspoon black pepper
½ teaspoon salt
12 cherry tomatoes, halved, or 4 plum
*   tomatoes, diced*
4 scallions, chopped
2 medium yellow or red bell peppers, seeded
*   and diced*
1 15-ounce can chickpeas, drained
¼ to ½ cup grated Parmesan cheese
6 to 8 large pieces leaf lettuce (optional)

In a large saucepan, place the pasta in enough boiling water to cover and cook for 10 to 12 minutes, until al dente. Drain and cool under cold running water.

Meanwhile, in a large mixing bowl, whisk together the oil, vinegar, mustard, garlic, herbs, and seasonings. Add the cooked pasta, tomatoes, scallions, peppers, and chickpeas and blend well. Fold in the Parmesan cheese. Chill for 1 hour before serving. Place over a bed of leaf lettuce.

Makes 4 to 6 servings

KITCHEN TIPS:
• Pepperoncini, a tingly Italian pepper, makes a delightful addition to the salad. They are sold in the Italian section of grocery stores. Chop up 2 or 3 and add to the salad.

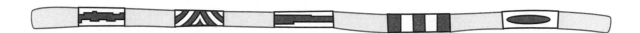

PEPPERY QUINOA AND MIXED BEAN SALAD

Are you in the mood for something completely different? Then try this piquant combination of exotic grains, beans, and vegetables.

1 cup quinoa, rinsed
2 cups water
1 15-ounce can black beans or red kidney beans, drained
2 to 3 scallions, chopped fine
2 tomatoes, cored and diced
1 medium green bell pepper, seeded and diced
1 to 2 jalapeño or Red Fresno peppers, seeded and minced
1 cup corn kernels, fresh or frozen
2 tablespoons canola oil
2 tablespoons red wine vinegar
2 teaspoons dried oregano
½ teaspoon ground cumin
½ teaspoon black pepper
½ teaspoon salt
1 lime, cut into 6 wedges
6 to 8 large pieces leaf lettuce or other greens (optional)

In a medium saucepan, add the quinoa and water and bring to a simmer. Cover and cook for about 15 minutes over medium heat, until all of the water is absorbed. Fluff and set aside for 5 minutes.

Meanwhile, in a large mixing bowl, combine the beans, scallions, tomatoes, peppers, corn, oil, vinegar, and seasonings. Blend in the cooked quinoa. Chill for about 1 hour.

Serve the salad over a bed of greens. Squeeze one wedge of lime over each serving at the table.

Makes 6 servings

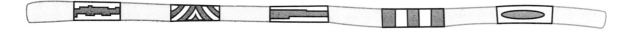

CUBAN BLACK BEAN AND RICE SALAD

I have an affinity for black beans and rice. The dynamic duo appears together in some of my favorite dishes, including Gallo Pinto and Brazilian Feijoada (see Index). Here they team up for this hearty Cuban-inspired salad.

2 15-ounce cans black beans, drained
2 cups cooked long-grain white or brown
    rice
4 scallions, chopped
2 medium tomatoes, diced
1 medium cucumber, peeled and diced
1 jalapeño or other chili pepper, seeded and
    minced (optional)
2 tablespoons canola oil
Juice of 1 lime
2 tablespoons chopped cilantro
2 teaspoons dried oregano
½ teaspoon ground cumin
½ teaspoon black pepper
½ teaspoon salt

In a large mixing bowl, combine the beans, rice, scallions, tomatoes, cucumber, and, if desired, jalapeño. Blend in the oil, lime juice, cilantro, and seasonings. Chill for about 1 hour before serving.

Makes 6 servings

KITCHEN TIPS
• For a slight twist, add 2 roasted, seeded, and chopped red bell peppers or (if available) New Mexico chili peppers.

FOUR-BEAN SALAD
FOR A CROWD

On my book-signing tour for *Lean Bean Cuisine*, I often brought this prodigious bean salad along to bookstores for customers to taste. Selling the book was easy once the customers sampled the salad. I find that this mélange of Mediterranean flavors appeals to a wide audience.

  1 15-ounce can white kidney beans, drained
  1 15-ounce can chickpeas, drained
  1 15-ounce can red kidney beans, drained
  1 15-ounce can black beans, drained
  2 medium red or green bell peppers, seeded and diced
  1 large cucumber, unpeeled and diced
  4 to 6 scallions, chopped
  2 large tomatoes, diced
  4 cloves garlic, minced
  ¼ cup rice vinegar or red wine vinegar
  ¼ cup olive oil
  2 tablespoons dried parsley (or 4 tablespoons chopped fresh)
  1 tablespoon dried oregano
  1 tablespoon dried mint or basil (or 2 tablespoons chopped fresh)
  2 teaspoons dried thyme leaves
  ½ teaspoon black pepper
  ½ teaspoon salt
  ¼ pound feta cheese, crumbled (optional)
  6 to 8 large pieces leaf lettuce (optional)

In a large mixing bowl, combine all of the ingredients (except lettuce) and blend thoroughly. Chill for at least 1 hour before serving.

Place in a large bowl with leaf lettuce arranged around the rim.

Makes 10 to 12 servings

WATERCRESS TABOULEH

Tabouleh is the ubiquitous wheat garden salad of Middle Eastern origins. My grandmother, who made tabouleh long before it was fashionable, supplied the inspiration for this recipe.

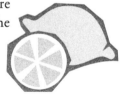

1 cup fine bulgur (cracked wheat)
2 cups boiling water
2 scallions, chopped fine
½ cup chopped parsley
¼ cup watercress leaves or 2 tablespoons
  chopped fresh mint
4 plum tomatoes, chopped
1 medium cucumber, peeled and chopped
Juice of 1 to 2 lemons
2 to 4 tablespoons olive oil
½ teaspoon black pepper
½ teaspoon salt
6 to 8 large pieces leaf lettuce or other leafy
  greens (optional)

In a medium saucepan, combine the bulgur and boiling water, cover, and let sit for 30 minutes to 1 hour, until all of the water is absorbed.

In a medium mixing bowl, combine the bulgur with the remaining ingredients (except lettuce) and toss thoroughly. Chill for at least 1 hour before serving. Place over a bed of leafy greens with warm pita bread.

Makes 4 servings

BEET AND RAISIN COLESLAW

Beets in coleslaw? This vivid adaptation of a traditional salad showcases the versatility and aesthetic qualities of beets. This is not really such a radical idea since raw beets appear in salads throughout the world. In this case the coleslaw turns purple, an added bonus! The kids will love it.

2 cups shredded green cabbage
2 cups scrubbed, shredded raw beets (about
  2 beets)
1 cup peeled, shredded carrots
¾ cup fat-free coleslaw dressing
2 tablespoons plain low-fat yogurt
½ cup dark raisins
½ teaspoon black pepper
½ teaspoon salt

In a large mixing bowl, combine all of the ingredients and blend thoroughly. Chill for at least 1 hour before serving.

Makes 4 to 6 servings

PEAR, ARUGULA, AND SWISS CHARD SALAD

The pear is almost as versatile as the apple; here it lends an intriguing touch to this simply prepared salad of wintry greens. A few drops of balsamic vinegar or rice vinegar complete the picture.

> 1 large bunch arugula (about 6 to 8 ounces)
> 10 to 12 leaves red Swiss chard, torn
> 2 plum tomatoes, quartered
> 2 medium carrots, peeled and sliced
> ½ medium unpeeled cucumber, sliced
>   (peeled only if waxed)
> ¼ cup crumbled feta cheese
> 2 to 3 Bosc pears, cored and sliced thin
> ¼ cup chopped hazelnuts or walnuts
>   (optional)
> Balsamic vinegar or rice vinegar, to taste

Rinse the arugula and Swiss chard and pat dry with a paper towel. In a large bowl, toss with the remaining vegetables and feta cheese. Arrange the pears around the edge. If desired, sprinkle nuts over the top and lightly drizzle the vinegar over the greens before serving.

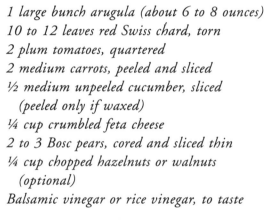

Makes 4 servings

KITCHEN TIPS:
* Kiwi Vinaigrette or Herb Dijon Vinaigrette (see Index) can also be served with Pear, Arugula, and Swiss Chard Salad.

COSTA RICAN CABBAGE SALAD

This Central American version of coleslaw, called *ensalada de repollo*, is lighter and more herbaceous than its North American counterpart. It is traditionally served with Gallo Pinto (see Index).

> 2 cups shredded white cabbage
> 1 large tomato, chopped
> 1 small cucumber, peeled and chopped
> 2 tablespoons minced cilantro
> 2 tablespoons minced parsley
> Juice of 1 lemon
> 1 tablespoon canola oil
> ½ teaspoon black pepper
> ½ teaspoon salt

In a medium mixing bowl, combine all of the ingredients and refrigerate for at least 30 minutes or, preferably, overnight. Serve the salad with a grain dish or a rice and bean dish.

Makes 4 servings

EMILY'S SPINACH AND SHREDDED BEET SALAD

My girlfriend Emily created this enterprising salad. Here the mundane spinach salad is transformed into a tantalizing first course. Shredded raw beets and jicama provide uplifting flavors and brilliant colors.

About ½ pound fresh spinach
2 to 3 plum tomatoes, quartered
1 medium fresh beet, scrubbed and shredded
1 large carrot, peeled and sliced thin
½ medium cucumber, sliced (peeled, if desired)
½ cup peeled, shredded jicama
2 large scallions, chopped
1 15-ounce can chickpeas, drained
1 cup washed and torn mizuna, frisee, or arugula leaves (optional)
2 ounces crumbled Gorgonzola cheese (optional)
½ cup Kiwi Vinaigrette or Herb Dijon Vinaigrette (see Index)

Rinse the spinach under cold running water. Drain, pat dry, and tear into bite-size pieces, removing the stems. Place in a large salad bowl. Add the tomatoes, beet, carrot, cucumber, jicama, scallions, chickpeas, and, if desired, mizuna and cheese and toss thoroughly.

Lightly drizzle the vinaigrette over the salad before serving. Serve with warm French bread.

Makes 4 servings

KITCHEN TIPS
- Mizuna is a tasty Japanese leaf that is available in Asian markets, natural food stores, and well-stocked supermarkets.

MESCLUN SALAD BOWL

Mesclun (the French term for "mixed field greens") is a collection of young leafy green vegetables. In the spring and summer, try a mixture of red leaf lettuce, watercress, arugula, mache, purslane, radicchio, young chard, and baby spinach. In autumn and winter, look for beet greens, mustard greens, dandelion greens, arugula, mizuna (a Japanese leaf), chard, and spinach. Small tender leaves make the best salad.

6 to 8 cups mixed rinsed and torn leafy greens
10 to 12 cherry tomatoes, halved
1 small red onion, slivered
1 small cucumber, sliced (peeled, if desired)
2 medium carrots, shredded
½ cup alfalfa or mung bean sprouts
Balsamic vinegar or your favorite dressing, to taste

In a large salad bowl, place the greens in the center and arrange the vegetables around the edge. Drizzle the vinegar over the top of the greens and vegetables. Serve with crusty French bread.

Makes 4 servings

MEXICAN BEAN SALAD WITH JICAMA, AVOCADO, AND LIME

This salad is replete with the earthy flavors and muted colors of legumes, avocados, and chilies. This is an opportunity to try an exotic Mexican chili such as ancho, a large dried poblano with a raisinlike flavor and subtle heat. Jicama (pronounced hee-cama) offers a crisp, water chestnutlike crunchiness.

1 15-ounce can black beans, drained
1 15-ounce can red kidney beans or pinto beans, drained
2 medium-size ripe avocados, peeled, pitted, and diced
2 large tomatoes, diced
1 cup peeled, diced jicama
2 large scallions, chopped
1 medium red or green bell pepper, seeded and diced
2 cloves garlic, minced
1 large ancho chili, soaked, drained, and minced
Juice of 1 lime
2 tablespoons chopped cilantro
2 teaspoons dried oregano

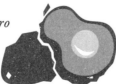

1 teaspoon ground cumin
½ teaspoon black pepper
½ teaspoon salt
6 to 8 large pieces leaf lettuce (optional)

In a large mixing bowl, combine all of the ingredients (except lettuce) and blend thoroughly. Chill for at least 1 hour before serving. Place over a bed of leaf lettuce.

Makes 6 servings

KITCHEN TIPS

- The dried ancho chili, available in Hispanic markets and well-stocked grocery stores, must be soaked in warm water for 30 minutes to 1 hour before using. If ancho chilies are unavailable, substitute a fresh serrano, jalapeño, or chipotle pepper.

COUSCOUS TROPICALE WITH BLACK BEANS AND CORN

I discovered this salad while visiting Key West, Florida, the southernmost tip of the country, where an outdoor restaurant called Mangoes served a lunch of couscous, black beans, and corn dressed lightly with a touch of a Key lime. I came home and made the salad with a regular lime, and the result was equally enticing.

1 cup couscous
1½ cups boiling water
2 medium tomatoes, diced
1 medium red or green bell pepper, seeded and diced
4 scallions, chopped
1 15-ounce can black beans, drained
2 cups corn kernels, fresh or frozen
2 tablespoons minced cilantro
½ teaspoon salt
½ teaspoon black pepper
Juice of 1 lime

In a medium bowl, combine couscous and boiling water, cover, and let stand for 10 minutes.

In a large mixing bowl, combine the couscous with the remaining ingredients; toss together thoroughly. Chill for 1 hour before serving.

Makes 4 to 6 servings

KITCHEN TIPS
• A Key lime tastes like a cross between a lime and a lemon. If it's available, you might use it instead of the regular lime.

GREEN BEAN AND POTATO SALAD WITH HERBES DE PROVENCE

Herbes de Provence is an aromatic blend of herbs grown in the French region of Provence. The mixture of dried thyme, sage, basil, rosemary, oregano, lavender, and mint offers a potpourri of fragrant flavors. This is just one of the many dishes that Herbes de Provence can enlighten.

4 cups unpeeled, diced Yukon gold or red potatoes
½ pound green beans, cut into 1-inch sections
⅓ cup plain low-fat yogurt
1 tablespoon Dijon-style mustard
2 to 3 teaspoons Herbes de Provence
½ teaspoon black pepper
½ teaspoon salt
1 cup finely chopped celery
4 scallions, chopped
6 to 8 large pieces leaf lettuce (optional)

In a medium saucepan, place the potatoes in enough boiling water to cover, and cook for about 15 minutes, until easily pierced with a fork. Drain and cool under cold running water.

In a medium saucepan, place the green beans in boiling water for about 4 minutes. Drain and cool under cold running water. (You may also steam the vegetables until tender.)

In a large mixing bowl, combine the yogurt, mustard, and seasonings. Add the potatoes, green beans, celery, and scallions and toss thoroughly. Chill for 1 hour before serving. Place over a bed of leaf lettuce.

Makes 4 servings

KITCHEN TIPS
- Herbes de Provence can be found in the spice section of well-stocked grocery stores.

THAI CUCUMBER SALAD

This spicy, palate-searing salad makes an exotic first course.

> *2 large unpeeled cucumbers, shredded*
> *1 red Thai chili or jalapeño, seeded and*
> *minced*
> *1 clove garlic, minced*
> *1 tablespoon light soy sauce*
> *Juice of 1 lime*
> *2 tablespoons chopped basil*
> *1 teaspoon brown sugar*

In a small mixing bowl, combine all of the ingredients and toss lightly. Refrigerate for at least 1 hour to allow the flavors to meld together.

Before serving, drain off some of the excess liquid.

Makes 4 servings

KITCHEN TIPS
- Thai chilies, also called bird peppers, are available in Asian markets. They have a sharp, prickly heat.

WARM POTATO AND PARSNIP SALAD WITH PEPPERCORN-MUSTARD DRESSING

If you are unfamiliar with parsnips, this is a good opportunity to start cooking with them. Parsnips lend a starchy sweetness to this piquantly flavored salad.

> *2 cups unpeeled, diced white potatoes*
> *2 cups peeled, diced parsnips*
> *2 tablespoons olive oil*
> *2 tablespoons red wine vinegar*
> *2 tablespoons Dijon-style mustard*
> *1 tablespoon prepared horseradish*
> *¼ cup minced fresh parsley (or 2 tablespoons*
> *dried)*
> *2 teaspoons black peppercorns, crushed*
> *(or 1 teaspoon coarse-ground black pepper)*
> *½ teaspoon salt*
> *2 scallions, chopped*
> *1 cup finely chopped celery*
> *1 small red onion, chopped fine*
> *6 to 8 large pieces leaf lettuce (optional)*

In a medium saucepan, place the potatoes in enough boiling water to cover, and cook for about 15 minutes, until tender. Drain and cool under cold running water.

In a medium saucepan, place the parsnips in enough boiling water to cover, and cook for 15

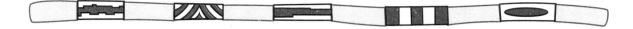

to 20 minutes, until tender. Drain and cool under cold running water.

In a large mixing bowl, combine the oil, vinegar, mustard, horseradish, parsley, peppercorns, and salt. Blend in the scallions, celery, onion, potatoes, and parsnips. Serve warm or chill for 1 hour. Serve over a bed of leaf lettuce.

Makes 4 servings

KITCHEN TIPS

- When they're in season, try dill, marjoram, or tarragon in place of (or in addition to) the parsley.

ASIAN PASTA SALAD WITH SPICY PEANUT SAUCE

In Japanese cuisine, thin white strands of somen noodles are often used in cold dishes. In this recipe, a peanut dressing coats the noodles with a savory nutty flavor. Rice vermicelli, another thin pasta popular in parts of Southeast Asia, may also be used.

½ *pound somen noodles or rice vermicelli*
¼ *cup chunky peanut butter*
¼ *cup hot water*
1 *tablespoon light soy sauce*
1 *tablespoon rice vinegar*
1 *teaspoon sesame oil*
1 *teaspoon hot sesame oil*
2 *cloves garlic, minced*
1 *Red Fresno or jalapeño chili pepper, seeded and minced*
4 *scallions, chopped fine*
6 to 8 *large pieces leaf lettuce (optional)*

In a medium saucepan, place the noodles in enough boiling water to cover, and cook for 3 to 5 minutes, until al dente. Drain and cool under cold running water.

In a medium mixing bowl, whisk together the peanut butter, water, soy sauce, rice vinegar, and sesame oils. Blend in the garlic and chili pepper. Toss the noodles with the peanut dressing. Chill for about 30 minutes before serving. Place the noodles on a bed of lettuce and top with the scallions.

Makes 3 to 4 servings

EGYPTIAN FAVA BEAN SALAD

The salads of the Middle East often rely on the triumvirate of lemon, parsley, and olive oil. In Egypt, this fava bean salad makes a popular lunch or first course. Look for small brown fava beans, which are available in natural food stores and well-stocked supermarkets. If you cannot find fava beans, try red chili beans or black-eyed peas instead.

2 15-ounce cans small fava beans, drained
2 medium tomatoes, diced
1 medium cucumber, peeled and diced
2 scallions or 1 small red onion, chopped
2 to 3 cloves garlic, minced
2 tablespoons olive oil
Juice of 1 lemon
¼ cup chopped parsley
½ teaspoon black pepper
¼ teaspoon salt
6 to 8 large pieces leaf lettuce (optional)

In a large mixing bowl, combine all of the ingredients (except lettuce) and toss together thoroughly. Chill for 1 hour before serving. Place over a bed of green leaf lettuce with warm pita bread on the side.

Makes 6 to 8 servings

KITCHEN TIPS
- Toss mint or cilantro leaves in with the salad, if desired.

SEASON'S FINEST TOMATO AND CHICKPEA SALAD

My grandparents grew them, my parents grew them, and I grow them. I'm talking about big, luscious, fire-engine red tomatoes. When the season is in full bloom, I walk out to the garden in the morning, pluck a ripe tomato from the vine, and bite into it like an apple. As far as I'm concerned, there's no better way to celebrate a new day.

There are so many ways to appreciate garden tomatoes at their finest. For this simple salad, fresh basil and parsley accentuate the tomatoes' summery flavor and chickpeas add nuttiness.

3 tablespoons olive oil
2 tablespoons red wine vinegar or balsamic vinegar
1½ teaspoons Dijon-style mustard
2 tablespoons chopped parsley
2 tablespoons chopped fresh basil (or 1 tablespoon dried)
½ teaspoon black pepper
¼ teaspoon salt
1 15-ounce can chickpeas, drained
4 to 6 medium-size ripe tomatoes, diced
1 medium yellow bell pepper, seeded and diced
2 large scallions, chopped

In a large mixing bowl, whisk together the oil, vinegar, mustard, herbs, and seasonings. Blend in the chickpeas, tomatoes, bell pepper, and scallions. Chill for 1 hour before serving.

Makes 6 servings

KITCHEN TIPS
- Sprigs of mint or oregano can also be added.

ROASTED BEET SALAD WITH DILL-HORSERADISH VINAIGRETTE

Roasting is an easy and flavor-enhancing way to cook beets. Simply wrap them in foil and bake them as you would a potato. Once cooked, the beets are ready to be chopped and tossed with a light dressing. For this salad, dill and horseradish accentuate the beets without overpowering their subtle flavor.

6 to 8 medium beets, scrubbed and rinsed
3 to 4 tablespoons canola oil
3 tablespoons red wine vinegar
2 teaspoons prepared horseradish
1 teaspoon Dijon-style mustard
1 teaspoon brown sugar, packed
2 tablespoons chopped parsley
1 tablespoon chopped dill
1 tablespoon chopped basil
½ teaspoon black pepper
½ teaspoon salt

Preheat the oven to 375°F.

Wrap the beets in aluminum foil and place on a baking pan. Roast for 50 minutes to 1 hour, until the beets are tender. Remove the beets from the oven, unwrap, and let cool.

Meanwhile, in a medium mixing bowl, whisk together the oil, vinegar, horseradish, mustard, brown sugar, herbs, and seasonings.

When the beets are cool enough to handle, peel off any blemishes or loose skin. Coarsely chop the beets and add to the vinaigrette; coat thoroughly. Let stand for 30 minutes and serve warm, or chill.

Makes 4 to 6 servings

KITCHEN TIPS
- Red-and-white sugar cane beets and orange beets can also be used.

CARIBBEAN HEAT SALAD

Sometimes I find a culinary treasure in the most out-of-the-way place. While conducting "field research" for my cookbook, *A Taste of the Tropics*, I discovered this unique dinner salad on St. John's, a quaint Caribbean island. The greens are cooked slightly in a dressing that has been infused with a fiery hot Scotch bonnet pepper. For my chili-friendly taste buds, this was the right side of paradise.

3 tablespoons canola oil
2 tablespoons red wine vinegar
1 teaspoon Dijon-style mustard
1 whole Scotch bonnet pepper, punctured with a fork
4 whole cloves
8 to 10 large Romaine leaves, torn into bite-size pieces
6 to 8 button mushrooms, sliced
½ small unpeeled cucumber, sliced
2 to 3 scallions, chopped
4 to 6 cherry tomatoes, halved
Salt and black pepper, to taste

In a large skillet, heat the oil, vinegar, and mustard. Add the Scotch bonnet pepper and cloves and cook for about 4 minutes over medium heat, stirring occasionally. Remove the cloves and add the greens, mushrooms, cucumber, and scallions and cover the pan. Cook for 3 to 5 minutes more, stirring occasionally, until the greens are wilted. Add the tomatoes and cook for 1 minute more.

Transfer the salad to serving plates. Remove the Scotch bonnet, cut into strips, discard seeds, and serve to those who savor hot food. Season the wilted greens with salt and pepper to taste.

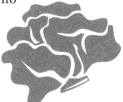

Makes 2 to 3 servings

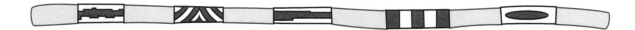

MIDDLE EASTERN BREAD SALAD (FETTOOSH)

My grandmother, a masterful cook for most of her eighty-plus years, never writes down her recipes. She talked me through this one: "When you don't feel like cooking much, you cook fettoosh. Take your leftover bread, cut it into small pieces, and fry it with an onion and squeeze lemon over it. Add a cucumber and tomato if you want. And don't forget the parsley."

2 tablespoons olive oil
1 medium yellow onion, diced (or 2
*   scallions, chopped)*
2 cups diced pita bread
2 medium tomatoes, diced
1 medium unpeeled cucumber, chopped
¼ cup chopped parsley
Juice of 1 lemon
½ teaspoon black pepper
½ teaspoon salt

In a skillet, heat the oil. Add the onion and cook over medium heat for 5 minutes. Add the bread and cook for 5 to 7 minutes more, stirring frequently.

Transfer the bread mixture to a medium salad bowl and toss with the remaining ingredients. Serve immediately.

Makes 4 servings

TUSCAN BREAD SALAD (PANZANELLA)

Panzanella is the name of the bread salad made famous in Tuscany. Here, stale bread is reincarnated as a salad; it is toasted and tossed together with tomatoes, fresh basil, olive oil, and vinegar. I prefer using day-old pumpernickel bread, but any dark bread will do.

4 to 5 slices pumpernickel bread
2 medium-size ripe tomatoes, diced
2 pepperoncini or other hot pickled peppers,
*   seeded and minced*
2 tablespoons olive oil
1 tablespoon balsamic vinegar
2 cloves garlic, minced
¼ cup chopped basil, parsley, or oregano
2 to 3 ounces part-skim mozzarella cheese,
*   cubed (optional)*
Salt and black pepper, to taste

Heat the oven to 300°F.

Place the bread on a baking pan and bake for 15 to 20 minutes, until lightly toasted. Cut the bread into bite-size squares.

In a mixing bowl, combine the remaining ingredients and the toasted bread and toss until blended thoroughly. Let stand for at least 15 minutes before serving.

Makes 2 to 3 servings

ZUCCHINI AND JICAMA SALAD WITH CHIPOTLE-LIME DRESSING

Every summer I look for new ways to cook with the truckload of summer squash that finds its way to my kitchen. This combination of zucchini, corn, jicama, and watercress makes a delightful salad for a picnic or outdoor barbecue. If you are looking for an alternative to coleslaw, give this south-of-the-border salad a taste.

1 medium zucchini, diced
1 medium yellow summer squash, diced
2 medium carrots, peeled and diced
1 cup peeled, diced jicama (about ½ pound)
1 cup corn kernels, fresh or frozen and
*   thawed*
Juice of 1 lime
2 tablespoons canola oil
1 canned chipotle pepper, seeded and minced
¼ cup watercress leaves or 2 tablespoons
*   chopped cilantro*
¼ teaspoon ground cumin
Salt, to taste
6 to 8 large pieces leaf lettuce (optional)

In a mixing bowl, combine all of the ingredients (except lettuce). Chill for about 30 minutes before serving. Place over a bed of leaf lettuce.

Makes 4 servings

KITCHEN TIPS

- For a barbecued salad, cut the squash in half lengthwise and grill over an open fire. Corn can also be grilled on the cob before adding to the salad.

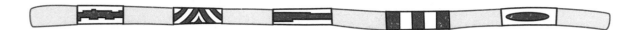

ORZO SALAD WITH MEDITERRANEAN FLAVORS

Orzo, also called rosa marina, is a small, rice shaped pasta that's ideal for light salads. Here it is adorned with Mediterranean herbs and spices.

½ pound orzo
3 tablespoons olive oil
2 tablespoons red wine vinegar
1 teaspoon Dijon-style mustard
¼ cup chopped fresh mint leaves (or 1½ tablespoons dried)
2 teaspoons dried oregano
1 teaspoon dried thyme leaves
½ teaspoon black pepper
2 medium tomatoes, diced
4 scallions, chopped
1 medium unpeeled cucumber, diced
2 cloves garlic, minced
1 cup pitted medium black olives, halved
¼ pound crumbled feta cheese
1 15-ounce can chickpeas, drained (optional)
6 to 8 large pieces leaf lettuce (optional)

In a small saucepan, place the pasta in boiling water and cook for 9 to 11 minutes, until al dente. Drain and cool under cold running water.

In a small bowl, whisk together the oil, vinegar, mustard, mint, and seasonings, forming a vinaigrette. In a large mixing bowl, combine the orzo, tomatoes, scallions, cucumber, garlic, and black olives. Blend in the vinaigrette, feta cheese, and, if desired, chickpeas. Chill for 1 hour before serving. Place over a bed of lettuce.

Makes 6 servings

GRILLED TUNISIAN VEGETABLE SALAD (SALATA MESHIWAYA)

Grilled vegetable salads are favorite dishes in Tunisia and other North African countries. The vegetables are delicately flavored with lemon, olive oil, and a touch of cumin and capers. "Salata Meshiwaya" means "salad cooked" or "barbecued salad." Couscous makes a perfect accompaniment.

2 tablespoons olive oil
Juice of 1 lemon
2 cloves garlic, minced
2 tablespoons minced parsley
1 tablespoon capers, rinsed and drained
¼ teaspoon ground cumin
2 medium green bell peppers, seeded and halved
2 medium red bell peppers, seeded and halved
2 large tomatoes, halved
1 medium red onion, peeled and quartered
1 jalapeño or other hot chili pepper, seeded and halved (optional)
4 to 5 cups cooked couscous (optional)

Preheat the grill until the coals are gray to white.

In a large mixing bowl, combine the olive oil, lemon juice, garlic, parsley, capers, and cumin. Set aside.

Place the vegetables and chili pepper on the grill. Cook for 7 to 10 minutes, occasionally turning, until the vegetables are tender (not charred).

Remove the vegetables and chili from the grill and place on a cutting board. Using a butter knife, scrape off and discard any charred parts. Coarsely chop all of the vegetables, mince the chili, and toss together with the oil-lemon mixture. Let sit for 10 to 15 minutes before serving. If desired, spoon the couscous onto serving plates and place the grilled vegetables on top.

Makes 3 to 4 servings

KITCHEN TIPS
- For a cross-cultural spin-off, substitute 2 New Mexico chilies for 2 of the bell peppers. New Mexico chilies have a piquant, fruity flavor and resilient flesh, and are perfect for grilling.
- For another version of fusion cuisine, grill a portobello mushroom (about ½ pound) and add it to the vegetable mix.

MINTY MIXED FRUIT SALAD

It used to be fashionable to bury fresh fruit in an avalanche of heavy cream and sugar. Thankfully, those days are history. A light yogurt dressing scented with mint is a far more eloquent (and healthful) way to extol the virtues of fresh fruit.

1 medium-size ripe cantaloupe
1 cup whole blueberries
1 cup strawberries, halved
3 kiwifruit, peeled and sliced
2 medium bananas, sliced
1 cup plain or vanilla nonfat yogurt
2 to 3 tablespoons chopped mint
1 tablespoon honey
½ teaspoon nutmeg or allspice
4 to 6 mint leaves (optional)

Cut the cantaloupe in half and scoop out and discard the seeds. With a melon ball scooper, scoop out the flesh, leaving the shells intact. (Set the shells aside for later.) In a large mixing bowl, combine the cantaloupe with the remaining ingredients. Chill until ready to serve.

For a fancy presentation, spoon the salad into the reserved cantaloupe shells. Garnish with extra mint leaves.

Makes 4 to 6 servings

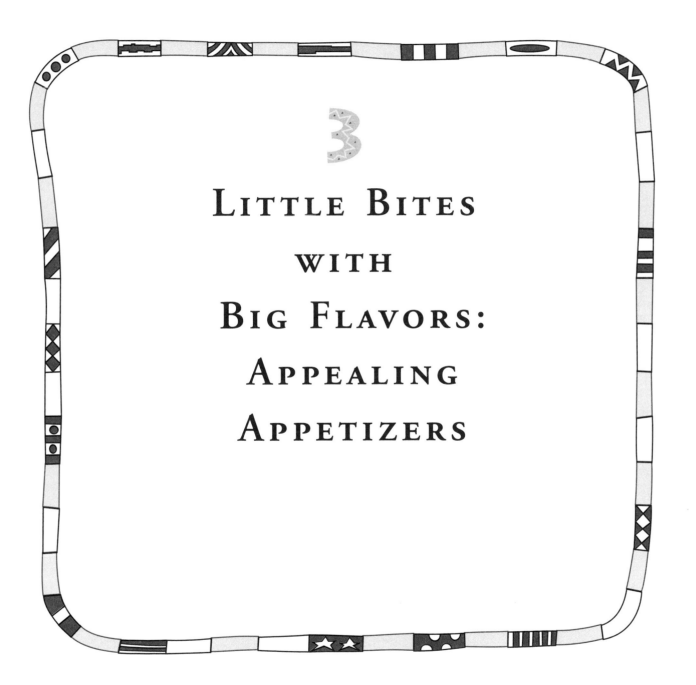

3

LITTLE BITES
WITH
BIG FLAVORS:
APPEALING
APPETIZERS

An appetizer should stimulate the appetite in small and unexpected ways; the palate should be pleasantly piqued. An appetizer should not be so filling and plentiful that it steals the thunder from the main course. Nor should it assault the palate with overpowering flavors of any sort, salty or otherwise. An appetizer's role is to make small talk with the taste buds until the big presentation arrives and takes over.

This chapter includes a stellar cast of small dishes, finger foods, and dips. Two all-time favorite recipes of mine, Sweet Potato Dal and Hawaiian Papaya Guacamole, head the list. There are also Middle Eastern Spinach Pies, Pimiento Polenta, Hummus with Roasted Red Chilies, and other appealing choices. These light bites will open the show with much aplomb and spirited flavors, but without upstaging the main act.

SWEET POTATO DAL

Dal is a classic Indian legume dish spiced with turmeric, cumin, and other warm curry flavors. It is important to cook the dal until it reaches a smooth, melt-in-your-mouth consistency.

1½ tablespoons canola oil
1 medium yellow onion, chopped fine
2 cloves garlic, minced
½ teaspoon turmeric
½ teaspoon ground cumin
½ teaspoon coriander or garam masala
¼ teaspoon black pepper
1 cup brown or red lentils, rinsed
4 cups water
2 cups peeled, diced sweet potatoes or
  butternut squash
½ teaspoon salt

In a saucepan, heat the oil. Add the onion and garlic and sauté for 5 minutes. Stir in the turmeric, cumin, coriander, and pepper; cook for 1 minute more. Stir in the lentils and water and cook over medium-low heat for 15 minutes, stirring occasionally. Stir in the potatoes and cook for about 30 minutes more, stirring occasionally, until the lentils are tender. Stir in the salt.

Transfer to a large serving bowl. Serve with an Indian flat bread or flour tortilla and Cucumber Cool Down (see Index).

Makes 4 to 6 servings

KITCHEN TIPS
- For a little more spice, sauté a minced chili pepper with the onion and garlic.
- Garam masala is a fragrant blend of spices available in Indian and natural foods stores and spice sections of well-stocked supermarkets.

HUMMUS WITH ROASTED RED CHILIES

Just when you thought that hummus had become a cliché—predictable and uninspiring—Pow! Along comes this spirited recipe. Roasted New Mexico red chilies reinvigorate hummus with a feel-good level of heat and a wallop of flavor.

> 2 fresh New Mexico red chilies
> 1 15-ounce can chickpeas, drained
> ½ cup plain low-fat yogurt
> ¼ cup tahini (sesame seed paste)
> Juice of 1 lemon
> 2 cloves garlic, minced
> ½ teaspoon ground cumin
> ¼ teaspoon black pepper
> ¼ teaspoon salt
> 2 tablespoons minced parsley

Roast the chilies by placing them over a hot grill or beneath a broiler for 4 to 6 minutes, occasionally turning, until the skin is charred. Remove the chilies from the heat and let cool for a few minutes. With a butter knife (or your hands), scrape and discard the charred skin from the flesh. Remove the seeds and chop the flesh.

Place the peppers and remaining ingredients (except the parsley) in a food processor fitted with a steel blade (or a blender) and process for about 15 seconds, until smooth. Transfer to a serving bowl and garnish with the parsley. Serve with warm pita bread and raw vegetables such as carrots, celery, sweet peppers, and broccoli.

Makes about 2 cups

KITCHEN TIPS
- There is no real substitute for New Mexico chilies, but roasted bell peppers can be used in a pinch or for a variation.
- This hummus also makes a tasty sandwich spread.

ROASTED EGGPLANT AND TAHINI DIP

This smoky eggplant dip, also called baba ghanoush, is rooted in Israeli cuisine. Once eggplant has been roasted or grilled, it becomes tender and pulpy, like a ripe avocado, and achieves a perfect consistency for dips and spreads. I like to spice the dip with a variety of fresh herbs. The eggplant can be broiled or grilled.

2 medium eggplants, cut in half lengthwise
2 cloves garlic, minced
¼ cup tahini (sesame seed paste)
2 to 3 tablespoons chopped parsley
2 tablespoons chopped mint (optional)
½ teaspoon ground cumin
¼ teaspoon black pepper
¼ teaspoon salt
Juice of 1 to 2 lemons

If broiling, place the eggplant face down on a baking pan. Preheat the broiler and, when ready, roast the eggplant beneath the heat until the skin crackles when touched and the flesh is tender. If grilling, grill the eggplant over an open fire for 7 to 10 minutes on each side, until the skin chars and the flesh is tender. Let cool slightly.

Meanwhile, in a mixing bowl, combine the remaining ingredients. Set aside until the eggplant is ready.

When the eggplant has cooled, peel off and discard the black skin. Coarsely chop the flesh and add to the tahini mixture. Place the mixture in a blender or a food processor fitted with a steel blade and process until smooth. (For a chunky consistency, mash the mixture with the back of a spoon.)

Serve warm or chilled as a vegetable dip, sandwich spread, or with pita bread.

Makes 4 to 6 servings

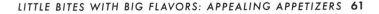

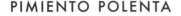

PIMIENTO POLENTA

Polenta is a down-to-earth dish with a high-society name. There are versions of this dense cornmeal cake in African, Caribbean, and Native American cuisines. The key is to add the cornmeal to the boiling water gradually to avoid clumping and to cook until a wooden spoon stands erect in the center of the mixture.

2½ cups water
½ teaspoon salt
¼ teaspoon black pepper
1 cup yellow fine cornmeal
2 tablespoons chopped pimiento
¼ cup grated Parmesan or Romano cheese
Vegetable spray
1 15-ounce can tomato sauce, heated

Combine the water, salt, and pepper in a small saucepan and bring to a boil. Very gradually stir in the cornmeal. Cook for 12 to 15 minutes over low heat, stirring frequently, until thick. Remove from the heat and fold in the pimiento and cheese. Spread the polenta in a lightly sprayed 9-inch round pan. Allow it to reach room temperature (about 15 minutes).

Cut the polenta into wedges. Place on serving plates and top with tomato sauce. If desired, serve with Tuscan White Beans (see Index).

Makes 6 to 8 servings

BABY BEETS IN YOGURT MARINADE

This dish is a popular appetizer in Eastern European and Middle Eastern countries. This Lebanese version calls for young, tender baby beets.

16 to 20 baby beets, scrubbed
2 cups plain low-fat yogurt
4 scallions, chopped
2 tablespoons minced parsley
½ teaspoon ground cumin
½ teaspoon black pepper
½ teaspoon salt

In a medium saucepan, place the beets in enough boiling water to cover and cook for 35 to 40 minutes, until tender. (Or wrap the beets in foil and roast in a 375°F oven for 45 minutes to 1 hour.) Drain the beets and cool slightly under cold running water.

In a medium mixing bowl, combine the yogurt, scallions, parsley, and spices. Fold the beets into the yogurt mixture and chill for at least 1 hour before serving.

Makes 4 servings

CROSTINI WITH SUN-DRIED TOMATOES AND ESCAROLE

Crostini means "little crusts" in Italian. It's an inventive way to use up yesterday's bread. Topped with sun-dried tomatoes and escarole, these open-faced sandwiches will stimulate your appetite for the meal to come.

> ½ cup sun-dried tomatoes (not oil packed)
> 1½ tablespoons olive oil
> 2 cloves garlic, minced
> 4 cups coarsely chopped, packed escarole or spinach
> ¼ teaspoon sage
> ¼ teaspoon red pepper flakes
> 8 thick slices Italian bread, toasted
> 2 tablespoons grated Parmesan cheese (optional)

Soak the tomatoes in enough warm water to cover for 30 minutes to 1 hour. Drain and chop coarse.

In a medium saucepan, heat the oil over medium heat. Add the garlic and sauté for 3 minutes. Stir in the tomatoes, escarole, and seasonings and cook for 3 to 4 minutes more, stirring frequently.

Spread the mixture over the toasted bread slices. If desired, sprinkle a little Parmesan cheese over the top of each slice.

Makes 8 servings

MIDDLE EASTERN SPINACH PIES

Although the world's cuisine is filled with empanadas, turnovers, and calzones, many are stuffed with some sort of meat. This authentic Middle Eastern recipe calls for a lemony spinach filling. For the dough, use one of your favorite bread recipes, or try a quality commercial bread or pizza dough from a local bakery.

1 10-ounce package fresh spinach
1 tablespoon olive oil
1 medium yellow onion, chopped fine
Juice of 1 lemon
½ teaspoon black pepper
½ teaspoon salt
1 pound chilled bread dough or pizza dough
Vegetable spray

Preheat the oven to 375°F.

Rinse the spinach under cold running water and remove the stems. Coarsely chop the leaves.

In a medium skillet, heat the oil. Add the onion and sauté for 2 to 3 minutes. Add the spinach, lemon, and seasonings and cook for 2 to 3 minutes more over low heat, until the spinach is wilted. Let cool slightly. Drain the excess liquid from the pan.

On a flat work surface, form the dough and divide into 8 equal balls. On wax paper or a floured surface, roll each ball into a flat circle.

Fill the center of each round with a few tablespoons of the spinach mixture. Fold the dough over the top of the filling and seal the edges with the back of a fork, forming a pocket. Place the pies onto a lightly sprayed baking pan and bake for 11 to 13 minutes, until golden brown.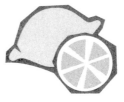

Remove from the heat and let cool for a few minutes before serving.

Makes 8 small pies

KITCHEN TIPS
- For a Greek variation, add 1 tablespoon of crumbled feta cheese to the spinach filling of each pie before sealing.

ARTICHOKES WITH PARSLEY TAHINI DIP

For those who cherish the artichoke, peeling its outer leaves is a labor of love. At the center of the artichoke, hidden beneath a mass of purple leaves and choke (a brushlike, bitter covering), lies the reward for one's efforts: the sumptuous heart. All that is needed now is a compatible dip, such as this herbed tahini offering.

1 cup plain low-fat yogurt
¼ cup tahini (sesame seed paste)
Juice of 1 lemon
2 cloves garlic, minced
¼ cup chopped parsley
½ teaspoon black pepper
½ teaspoon salt
4 whole artichokes, stems removed

To make the dip, in a small mixing bowl, whisk all of the ingredients (except the artichokes). Transfer to a serving bowl and refrigerate until ready to serve.

In a medium saucepan, place the artichokes in enough boiling water to cover. Boil for 35 to 45 minutes or until the artichoke bottoms are easily pierced with a fork. Remove the artichokes with tongs and place them upside down in a colander to drain.

Place each artichoke in a small bowl. Dip the leaves (one at a time) into the parsley-yogurt condiment.

Makes 4 servings

JAMAICAN JERK TEMPEH

The earthy, spicy characteristics of Jamaican jerk barbecue are a perfect match for the distinctive raw, untamed flavor of tempeh (a soybean product). This recipe first appeared in an article I wrote for *Vegetarian Times* magazine.

> *4 scallions, chopped*
> *1 small yellow onion, chopped*
> *1 teaspoon minced Scotch bonnet pepper or other chili pepper*
> *¼ cup light soy sauce*
> *¼ cup red wine vinegar*
> *2 tablespoons canola oil*
> *2 tablespoons brown sugar, packed*
> *1½ teaspoons dried thyme (or 1 tablespoon fresh)*
> *½ teaspoon nutmeg*
> *½ teaspoon allspice*
> *1 pound tempeh, cut into ½-inch squares*
> *6 to 8 large pieces leaf lettuce*

Preheat the oven to 375°F.

Combine all of the ingredients (except the tempeh) in a blender or a food processor fitted with a steel blade. Process the mixture for 10 to 15 seconds at high speed. Pour the sauce into a 9″ × 13″ casserole dish or baking pan. Place the tempeh in the pan and cover with the sauce.

Bake for 10 to 15 minutes, until the tempeh forms a brown crust.

To serve, remove the tempeh from the sauce and place on a serving plate lined with leaf lettuce. Scrape the remaining sauce into a small dish and offer as a dipping sauce.

Makes 8 servings

HAWAIIAN PAPAYA GUACAMOLE

When traveling, I have a penchant for cooking with local ingredients. I was in sunny Hawaii when I created this luscious tropical avocado dip with sweet island papayas.

> *2 medium-size ripe avocados, peeled, pitted, and chopped*
> *1 medium papaya, peeled, halved, seeded, and chopped*
> *1 large tomato, diced*
> *¼ cup finely chopped red onion*
> *2 cloves garlic, minced*
> *2 tablespoons minced cilantro*
> *Juice of 1 lime*
> *½ teaspoon ground cumin*
> *½ teaspoon salt*
> *½ teaspoon black pepper*
> *2 scallions, chopped*

Place all of the ingredients (except the scallions) in a food processor fitted with a steel blade and process for about 10 seconds. (Or, mash the ingredients by hand in a mixing bowl, forming a chunky paste.) Transfer to a serving bowl and top with the scallions. Serve with baked tortilla chips and raw vegetables.

Makes 4 to 6 servings

KITCHEN TIPS
- You can determine an avocado's ripeness by holding it in the base of your hand and pressing down lightly with your thumb; it should give a little bit.

GRILLED ANTIPASTO

Antipasto once meant a platter of limp, over-cooked vegetables. This improved version calls for grilled and lightly marinated vegetables. If you like to grill, you'll love preparing this dish.

¼ cup chopped basil or watercress
2 tablespoons olive oil
2 tablespoons balsamic vinegar or red wine vinegar
2 to 3 cloves garlic, minced

Vegetable spray
3 to 4 plum tomatoes
1 large portobello mushroom, sliced
1 large yellow onion, peeled and halved
2 medium red or green bell peppers, seeded and halved
1 medium eggplant, cut widthwise into thin ovals
1 medium zucchini, cut widthwise into thin ovals
2 to 3 ounces part-skim milk mozzarella cheese, cubed
Salt and black pepper, to taste

In a large mixing bowl, combine the basil, oil, vinegar, and garlic and set aside.

Preheat grill until the coals are gray to white.

Lightly spray the grill and place all of the vegetables on it. Cook for 7 to 10 minutes, turning after 5 minutes. When the tomatoes are ready to burst, pull them off and place them in the oil-and-vinegar mixture. Remove the remaining vegetables as they become tender and develop hatch marks, and place them in the bowl as well. Add the cheese and toss thoroughly. Let stand for a few minutes to allow the flavors to intermingle. Season with salt and pepper to taste. Serve with Italian bread.

Makes 4 servings

EGGPLANT AND CUCUMBER RAITA

This is a cross between Roasted Eggplant and Tahini Dip and Cucumber Cool Down (see Index). It is vastly more pleasurable (and more healthful) than the hackneyed French onion soup–sour cream concoctions that dominate the chip-and-dip circuit.

Vegetable spray
1 medium eggplant, cut in half lengthwise
1 cup plain low-fat yogurt
1 medium unpeeled cucumber, chopped fine
2 cloves garlic, minced
2 tablespoons tahini (sesame seed paste)
2 to 3 scallions, chopped
1 teaspoon ground cumin
½ teaspoon black pepper
½ teaspoon salt
Juice of 1 lemon

On a lightly sprayed baking pan, place the eggplant cut-side down. Roast the eggplant beneath a hot broiler for 7 to 10 minutes, until the skin "crackles" to the touch and the flesh is tender. Remove from the heat and let cool.

Meanwhile, in a medium mixing bowl, combine the remaining ingredients. Set aside until the eggplant is cool.

Peel off and discard the eggplant's skin. Coarsely chop the flesh and add to the yogurt mixture; blend thoroughly. Refrigerate for at least 30 minutes to allow the flavors to mingle.

Serve with vegetables or pita bread as a dip or use as a sandwich spread.

Makes 6 servings

PINTO BEAN AND CORN QUESADILLA

Quesadillas make a quick and easy appetizer for almost any occasion.

1½ cups corn kernels, fresh or frozen and thawed
1 15-ounce can pinto beans or black beans, drained
3 to 4 scallions, chopped
1 jalapeño pepper, seeded and minced
2 tablespoons minced cilantro
½ teaspoon ground cumin
½ teaspoon salt
8 6-inch flour tortillas
Vegetable spray
¼ pound low-fat Swiss cheese or low-fat provolone, sliced thin

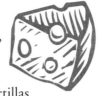

Preheat the oven to 400°F.

In a medium mixing bowl, combine the corn, beans, scallions, jalapeño, cilantro, and seasonings. Arrange 4 tortillas on 2 lightly sprayed baking pans. Spread an equal amount of the bean-corn mixture on top of each of the tortillas. Layer the cheese over each filling, and cover with the remaining tortillas. Place in the oven and bake for 7 to 10 minutes, until the tortillas are lightly browned.

Transfer the quesadillas to serving plates. Cut into wedges and serve with Salsa! Salsa!, Roasted Vegetable Salsa with Watercress, Hawaiian Papaya Guacamole (see Index for recipes), or your favorite salsa.

Makes 6 to 8 small servings

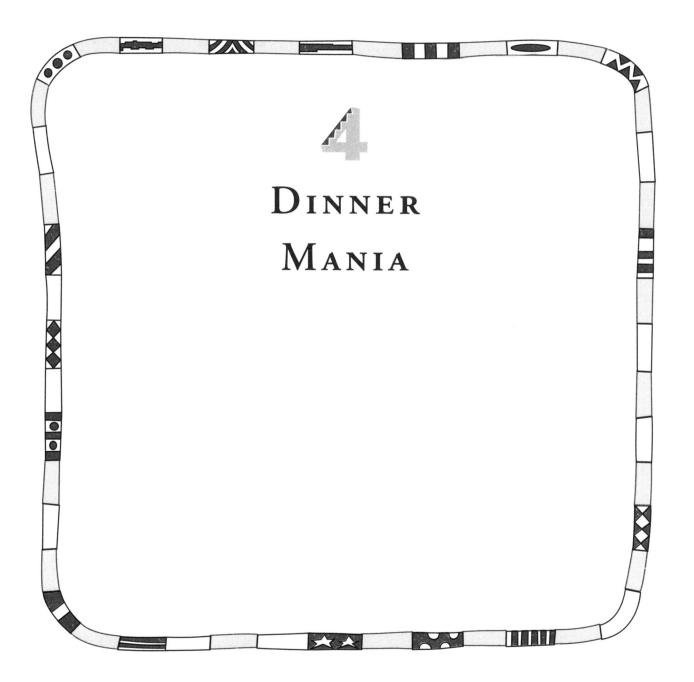

4

DINNER
MANIA

innertime is a special time. While breakfast is often eaten on the run and lunch is usually constrained by time and place, dinner revolves around the center of the plate. It is a time to replenish, reflect, and occasionally, even luxuriate. And for dinner, you want a winner.

To many cooks, however, dinner is the most daunting of meals to prepare, especially when it's a vegetarian dinner. While meatless soups and side dishes appear within one's reach, a meat-free main course can seem a bit more challenging. Yet with a little imagination and preparation, it is indeed possible to assemble a wide range of hearty meatless feasts.

The recipes in this chapter span the world and feature an eclectic selection of culturally diverse and healthful main entrees. From Pumpkin Risotto with Spinach and Vegetable Quinoa Bake to Garden Harvest Ratatouille and West African Jollof Rice, the menu crisscrosses the epicurean globe. There are Jamaican Jerk Vegetables, Spicy Squash and Chickpea Curry, South American Vegetable Stew, Bow-Tie Pasta with Italian Garden Vegetables, and much, much more. This is vegetarian cooking at its best.

For the meatless supper hour, vegetables, grains, and legumes share the limelight. There are squash galore—butternut, acorn, red kuri, and West Indian pumpkin. Potatoes, parsnips, carrots, eggplant, corn, peppers, and green leafy vegetables make frequent appearances. An international pantry of rices, couscous, bulgur, and barley, and all kinds of pastas and beans display their versatility. Distinctive spices and herbs lend depth and panache.

Here is proof that a meatless dinner need not be intimidating or cause for panic. It is a welcome opportunity to delight, satisfy, and at times, pleasantly surprise the palate.

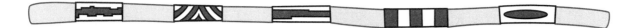

PUMPKIN RISOTTO WITH SPINACH

Risotto is a mellifluous Italian dish made with arborio rice, a short, pearly white grain. While most rice dishes yearn to be fluffy, risotto aspires to be creamy and dense. Pumpkin melds smoothly into this risotto and offers up a comforting taste of autumn. Butternut squash or red kuri squash also can be used.

1 tablespoon olive oil or canola oil
1 medium yellow onion, chopped fine
12 medium button mushrooms, sliced
2 cloves garlic, minced
2 cups peeled, diced sugar pumpkin or
  butternut or red kuri squash
2 cups arborio rice
1 cup peeled, diced carrots
1½ cups chopped fresh spinach or red Swiss
  chard
½ teaspoon white pepper
½ teaspoon salt
5 cups water
¼ cup plus 2 tablespoons grated Parmesan
  cheese

In a large saucepan, heat the oil. Add the onion, mushrooms, and garlic and sauté for about 7 minutes. Add the squash, rice, carrots, spinach, seasonings, and half of the water. Cook over medium-low heat for about 10 minutes, stirring frequently.

Add the remaining water and cook for 8 to 10 minutes more, stirring frequently. Turn off the heat and fold in the cheese. Let stand for 5 minutes. Serve the risotto with warm bread.

Makes 6 servings

CAULIFLOWER, LENTIL, AND SWEET POTATO CURRY

Indian cuisine is naturally meatless and energetically seasoned. Curry, India's vibrant national spice, brings out the best in these vegetables and legumes.

1 cup green lentils, rinsed
5 cups water
½ teaspoon turmeric
1 tablespoon canola oil
1 large yellow onion, diced
3 to 4 cloves garlic, minced
2 medium tomatoes, diced
1 tablespoon curry powder
2 teaspoons ground cumin
1 teaspoon salt
¼ teaspoon cayenne pepper
¼ teaspoon ground cloves
2 cups unpeeled, diced sweet potatoes
8 medium cauliflower florets
2 cups coarsely chopped kale, escarole, or spinach

In a medium saucepan, place the lentils, water, and turmeric and cook for about 45 minutes over medium-low heat. Set aside.

In a large saucepan, heat the oil. Add the onion and garlic and sauté over medium heat for 4 minutes. Add the tomatoes and sauté for 4 minutes more. Add the remaining seasonings, reduce the heat to low, and cook for 1 minute more, stirring frequently.

Stir the lentils, cooking liquid, potatoes, and cauliflower into the curry mixture. Cook for about 20 minutes over medium heat, stirring occasionally, until the potatoes and cauliflower are tender. Stir in the leafy greens and cook for 5 to 10 minutes more over low heat.

Serve over basmati or jasmine rice with Cucumber Cool Down (see Index) or plain low-fat yogurt with warm chapati (Indian bread) or another flat bread on the side.

Makes 4 servings

KITCHEN TIPS

- For a slight variation, substitute 1½ teaspoons of garam masala for the ground cumin. Adding ½ teaspoon ground fenugreek is also an option.
- Garam masala is a fragrant spice blend usually containing cumin, coriander, cardamom, and other spices. Fenugreek is a subtle aromatic spice found in Indian pantries. Both are available at Indian groceries and well-stocked natural food stores.

SUNDAY PILAF WITH PAN-ROASTED VERMICELLI AND CHICKPEAS

When I was growing up, almost every Sunday my family made the short trip to our grandmother's house in Myers, New York, a small ethnic village near Ithaca. Waiting for us on the stove top would be a large stockpot of roasted noodles, rice, and chickpeas called *shy-diaye*, or pilaf to the outside visitor.

This meatless adaptation is faithful to the spirit of the dish.

> *½ pound vermicelli or angel hair pasta*
> *2 tablespoons margarine or canola oil*
> *1 tablespoon olive oil*
> *1 medium yellow onion, chopped fine*
> *1 medium summer squash, diced*
> *1 medium green or red bell pepper, seeded and diced*
> *4 cups water*
> *1½ cups long-grain white rice or parboiled rice*
> *1 15-ounce can chickpeas, drained*
> *½ teaspoon turmeric*
> *½ teaspoon black pepper*
> *½ teaspoon ground cumin*
> *1 teaspoon salt*

Break up the vermicelli into small pieces over a large bowl.

In a large, deep skillet, heat the margarine. Add the uncooked vermicelli and cook over medium heat for about 10 minutes, stirring frequently. Remove the pan from the heat when the noodles are golden brown.

Meanwhile, in a large saucepan, heat the oil. Add the onion, squash, and bell pepper and sauté for about 7 minutes, until the vegetables are tender. Stir in the water, rice, chickpeas, seasonings, and roasted vermicelli. Cover the pan and cook over low heat for about 15 to 20 minutes, until all of the liquid is absorbed.

Fluff the pilaf and let stand for 5 to 10 minutes on the warm burner before serving.

Makes 6 to 8 servings

BAKED PUMPKIN WITH VEGETABLE PILAF

Pumpkin has long been unfairly stereotyped as either a pie filling or a Halloween ornament. In reality, it is much more versatile than people give it credit for. When baked and stuffed, pumpkin becomes a magnificent centerpiece. This vegetable pilaf is one of my favorite "stuffings," but you can fill a pumpkin with almost any grain dish. This recipe first appeared in an article I wrote for *Vegetarian Times* magazine.

> 1 5- to 6-pound pumpkin or red kuri
>   squash
> 1 tablespoon canola oil
> 1 small yellow onion, diced
> 1 medium red or green bell pepper, seeded
>   and diced
> 1 small jalapeño pepper, seeded and minced
> 1 small zucchini, diced
> 2 tablespoons minced shallots
> 1½ cups brown rice
> ¼ cup dark raisins
> ½ teaspoon black pepper
> ¼ teaspoon turmeric
> ¼ teaspoon salt
> 3 cups water
> 8 medium broccoli florets, blanched
> 2 tablespoons minced cilantro (optional)

Preheat the oven to 375°F.

With a sharp knife, cut a 4-inch-diameter lid off the top of the pumpkin. With a large spoon, scoop out the seeds and stringy fibers; discard them or save them for another use. Line the inside of the pumpkin with aluminum foil and set the pumpkin lid back on top. Place in a baking pan filled with ½-inch water and bake for 50 minutes to 1 hour, until the inside is tender. Remove from the heat and keep warm.

Meanwhile, make the pilaf. In a medium saucepan, heat the oil. Add the onion, peppers, zucchini, and shallots and sauté for about 7 minutes, until the vegetables are tender. Stir in the rice, raisins, and seasonings and cook for 1 minute more. Add the water. Cover and cook for about 45 minutes over medium-low heat, until the liquid is absorbed.

Fluff the pilaf and stir in the broccoli and cilantro. Remove the foil from the pumpkin. Spoon the pilaf into the center of the pumpkin and cover with the lid. Present the pumpkin on a large platter in the center of the table. When serving the pilaf, scrape the inside of the pumpkin with a spoon and mix the flesh into the rice.

Makes 4 servings

CREOLE EGGPLANT AND BLACK-EYED PEA STEW

A triumvirate of spices—black pepper, cayenne, and Tabasco—gives this vegetable stew a well-balanced level of heat. This is the kind of spirited Creole dish you might find in the Caribbean.

2 tablespoons olive oil
4 cups diced eggplant (about 1 medium eggplant)
2 large tomatoes, diced
1 medium yellow onion, diced
1 medium green bell pepper, seeded and diced
2 cloves garlic, minced
1 28-ounce can crushed tomatoes
1 cup water
1 tablespoon dried oregano
2 teaspoons dried thyme leaves
½ teaspoon black pepper
¼ teaspoon cayenne pepper
½ teaspoon salt
1 15-ounce can black-eyed peas or red kidney beans, drained
Tabasco or other bottled hot sauce, to taste

In a large saucepan, heat the oil. Add the eggplant, tomatoes, onion, bell pepper, and garlic and cook over medium heat for about 10 minutes, stirring frequently. Add the crushed tomatoes, water, and seasonings and cook over medium-low heat for 25 minutes, stirring occasionally. Stir in the black-eyed peas and Tabasco (to taste) and let stand for 10 minutes.

Serve with Bayou Red Beans, Pimiento Polenta (see Index for recipes), and brown rice. Pass the bottle of Tabasco at the table.

Makes 6 servings

SUCCOTASH-STUFFED BUTTERNUT SQUASH

Succotash, a traditional Native American dish of corn and beans, artfully fills this autumn squash. Butternut squash are the long, thin-skinned tan gourds with the bell-shaped end. This dish makes an attractive centerpiece to a meal.

2 medium butternut squash
2 cups baby green lima beans, fresh or
*   frozen*
1 tablespoon canola oil
1 medium red onion, diced
2 medium red or green bell peppers, seeded
*   and diced*
1 jalapeño pepper, seeded and minced
*   (optional)*
2 cloves garlic, minced
2 cups corn kernels, fresh or frozen
1½ teaspoons dried oregano
½ teaspoon dried thyme
½ teaspoon black pepper
¼ teaspoon nutmeg
¼ teaspoon salt
¼ cup bread crumbs
¼ cup grated Parmesan cheese

Preheat the oven to 350°F.

Cut the squash in half lengthwise. Scoop out and discard the seeds and stringy fibers. Place the squash cut-side down on a sheet pan filled with about ¼-inch water. Bake for 35 to 40 minutes, until the flesh is easily pierced with a fork. Remove from the oven, flip the squash over, drain the water from the pan, and let cool for a few minutes.

Meanwhile, in a small saucepan, place the lima beans in enough boiling water to cover and cook for 10 minutes. Drain and cool slightly.

In a medium saucepan, heat the oil. Add the onion, peppers, and garlic and sauté for 5 to 7 minutes. Add the lima beans, corn, and seasonings and cook over low heat for 5 minutes more, stirring occasionally. Remove from the heat and keep warm.

When the squash is cool, scoop out the flesh from the shells, coarsely chop, and blend into the succotash. Spoon the succotash back into the shells and sprinkle with bread crumbs and cheese. Place the stuffed squash beneath a hot broiler for 5 to 7 minutes, until lightly browned.

Present the stuffed squash on large serving platters at the table. Serve with Stove Top Quinoa Pilaf or Dandelion Rice and Sweet

Potatoes (see Index for recipes), or other grain dishes.

Makes 4 servings

JAVANESE NOODLES WITH PEANUT SAUCE

This recipe comes from Java, an Indonesian island known for dishes with peanut sauces. One key ingredient here is ketjap manis, a sweetened version of soy sauce. Rice sticks are thin, vermicellilike noodles that cook up quickly. This dish also tastes good cold, so make extra for tomorrow's lunch.

½ pound rice sticks (or rice vermicelli)
1 tablespoon peanut oil or canola oil
1 medium red bell pepper, seeded and chopped fine
1 serrano or other hot chili pepper, seeded and minced
2 cloves garlic, minced
1 tablespoon minced gingerroot
6 tablespoons chunky peanut butter
¼ cup hot water
3 tablespoons ketjap manis (or 3 tablespoons light soy sauce sweetened with 1 tablespoon brown sugar)
2 tablespoons lime juice
1 to 2 teaspoons sesame oil
5 to 6 scallions, chopped
2 tablespoons minced cilantro
8 to 10 broccoli florets, blanched (optional)

In a medium saucepan, place the rice sticks in boiling water and cook for 3 to 5 minutes, until al dente. Drain and set aside.

In a saucepan, heat the oil. Add the peppers, garlic, and gingerroot. Whisk in the peanut butter, water, ketjap manis, lime juice, and sesame oil. Bring the sauce to a simmer, stirring frequently. Remove from the heat and add the scallions and cilantro.

Place the noodles on serving plates and spoon the peanut sauce over the top. Garnish with the broccoli florets, if desired.

Makes 4 servings

KITCHEN TIPS
- Ketjap manis and rice sticks are available in the Asian section of well-stocked grocery stores and in Asian markets.
- Peppery arugula or Thai basil can be added in place of cilantro.

JAY'S VEGGIE BURRITO

For years I served this unintimidating dish at my restaurant. It topped the charts as one of the most all-time popular items on the menu. I encourage improvisation: add cashews, red beans, a few tablespoons of pesto, green peas, or whatever your palate desires.

1 tablespoon canola oil
1 small zucchini, diced or 1½ cups diced eggplant
6 to 8 medium button mushrooms, sliced
6 broccoli florets (preferably blanched)
1 medium green or red bell pepper, seeded and diced
½ cup corn kernels, fresh or frozen and thawed
½ teaspoon ground cumin
½ cup shredded low-fat provolone or Swiss cheese
2 10-inch flour tortillas, warmed

In a large skillet, heat the oil. Add the zucchini, mushrooms, broccoli, and pepper and cook over medium heat for 5 to 7 minutes, stirring occasionally, until the vegetables are tender. Reduce the heat to low and stir in the corn and cumin; cook for 2 to 3 minutes more. Remove from the heat and quickly blend in the cheese.

Place the warmed tortillas on plates and spoon the vegetable and cheese mixture into the center of each tortilla, forming a log. Wrap the tortillas around the vegetable mixture like a crepe, finishing with the seam-side down. Serve with Southwestern Green Rice and Salsa! Salsa! (see Index for recipes) or your favorite salsa.

Makes 2 large servings

CAPELLINI WITH ARRABIATA SAUCE

Arrabiata, which means "mad" or "enraged" in Italian lingo, is a spicy dish seasoned with red pepper flakes and pepperoncinis (pickled Italian hot peppers). The sauce is feisty and fluid, but rich enough to cling to the pasta. I include a lot of vegetables in my arrabiata.

2 tablespoons olive oil
1 medium yellow or green zucchini, diced
1 medium green bell pepper, seeded and diced
1 cup diced eggplant
2 cloves garlic, minced
2 to 3 pepperoncinis, seeded and minced
1 28-ounce can stewed tomatoes
1 28-ounce can tomato puree
2 tablespoons dried parsley
1 tablespoon dried basil
1 tablespoon dried oregano
¼ teaspoon red pepper flakes
½ teaspoon salt
¾ pound capellini or linguini
2 scallions, chopped fine

In a large saucepan, heat the oil. Add the zucchini, bell pepper, eggplant, and garlic and cook over medium heat for 7 to 10 minutes, stirring occasionally, until the vegetables are tender. Stir in the pepperoncinis, stewed tomatoes, tomato puree, and seasonings. Reduce the heat to low and simmer for 35 to 45 minutes, stirring occasionally. (Partially cover the pan to keep the sauce from splattering.)

Meanwhile, place the pasta in a large saucepan of boiling water, stir, and return to a boil. (I prefer to snap the noodles in half before cooking.) Cook according to package directions until al dente (4 to 6 minutes for capellini, 9 to 12 minutes for linguini). Drain and transfer to warm serving plates. Spoon the red sauce over the pasta and top with the scallions. Serve with warm bread.

Makes 6 servings

KITCHEN TIPS
- Pepperoncinis are available in the Italian pantry sections of most well-stocked grocery stores.
- If desired, add a few chopped basil leaves to the sauce a few minutes before serving.
- For an even spicier dish, add a chopped serrano or jalapeño pepper to the sauce.

BOW-TIE PASTA WITH ITALIAN GARDEN VEGETABLES

The kitchen garden plays a big role in Italian cooking, and this healthful dish was inspired by the bountiful Italian gardens I have known.

> 8 to 12 ounces bow-tie pasta
> 1 tablespoon olive oil
> 2 cloves garlic, minced
> 1 medium unpeeled green or yellow zucchini, diced
> 1 medium red or green bell pepper, seeded and diced
> 8 to 10 button mushrooms, sliced
> About 16 sweet cherry tomatoes, halved
> 2 cups coarsely chopped rapini, escarole, or chard
> 2 tablespoons chopped parsley
> 1 tablespoon chopped basil
> 1 tablespoon chopped oregano
> Black pepper and salt, to taste
> 2 to 3 tablespoons grated Parmesan or Romano cheese (optional)

In a large saucepan, place the pasta in boiling water, stir, and return to a boil. Cook according to package directions until al dente (about 9 to 12 minutes). Drain and place into a large bowl.

In a large skillet, heat the oil. Add the garlic, zucchini, pepper, and mushrooms and sauté for about 7 minutes. Stir in the tomatoes, rapini, and herbs. Cover and cook for about 4 minutes over medium heat, stirring frequently.

Add the vegetables to the pasta and toss together. Season with black pepper and salt and, if desired, grated Parmesan or Romano cheese at the table.

Makes 4 servings

KITCHEN TIPS

- Rapini, also called broccoli rabe, is a leafy green vegetable with a strong, mustardlike flavor. It is available in the produce section of well-stocked grocery stores.
- If desired, add a few leaves of arugula or mint along with the herbs. Or try a flavored pasta, such as parsley garlic, kamut spirals, or spinach noodles.
- If yellow cherry tomatoes are available, use in place of red cherry tomatoes.
- For a spicy delight, add a minced hot chili pepper along with the vegetables.

PENNE PRIMAVERA WITH PESTO REDUX

Traditional pesto, however heavenly, is often laden with oil and calories. For pesto redux, I've replaced most of the oil with a diced tomato, and still achieved the distinctive pesto aroma and flavor that everyone enjoys. While basil is the traditional herb for pesto, a mixture of garden herbs offers a refreshing change of pace. Toss it with penne and vegetables and a meal is born.

FOR THE PESTO:

4 cloves garlic
¼ cup diced walnuts or pine nuts
2 cups mixed herbs (any combination of
   basil, mint, oregano, and parsley)
1 large tomato, diced
¼ cup olive oil
½ teaspoon black pepper
½ teaspoon salt
¼ to ½ cup grated Parmesan cheese

FOR THE PASTA:

½ pound penne or ziti
1 medium red bell pepper, seeded and diced
About 16 sweet cherry tomatoes, halved
10 to 12 small broccoli florets, blanched

Add the garlic and nuts to a food processor fitted with a steel blade. Process for about 10 seconds, stopping once to scrape the sides. Add the herbs, tomato, oil, and seasonings and process for 10 seconds more, until smooth. Stop at least once to scrape the sides. Transfer to a mixing bowl and fold in the cheese. Set aside.

In a medium saucepan, place the pasta in enough boiling water to cover, stir, and return to a boil. Cook according to package directions (or until al dente, 9 to 12 minutes). Drain and place into a large serving bowl.

Add the pesto and vegetables to the pasta and toss together.

The pesto can be made earlier in the day and kept refrigerated until ready to serve with the vegetables and pasta.

Makes 4 servings

GARDEN HARVEST RATATOUILLE

When I plant my garden every spring, it seems I have ratatouille in mind. This crowd-pleaser is the Mediterranean stew of eggplant, tomatoes, summer squash, and other vegetables, many of which I valiantly attempt to grow.

1 tablespoon olive oil
1 large yellow onion, slivered
2 large cloves garlic, minced
1 medium green bell pepper, seeded and diced
2 cups diced eggplant (about 1 small eggplant)
1 medium summer squash, diced
4 medium-size ripe tomatoes, diced
1 tablespoon dried basil
1 tablespoon dried oregano
1 teaspoon salt
¼ teaspoon cayenne pepper
2 cups coarsely chopped beet greens, escarole, or other leafy greens
¼ cup grated Parmesan or Romano cheese

In a saucepan, heat the oil. Add the onion and sauté for 5 minutes. Add all of the remaining ingredients (except the greens and cheese) and cook over medium-low heat for 15 minutes, stirring occasionally. Stir in the greens and cook for about 5 minutes more.

Serve the stew over couscous, rice, or pasta and sprinkle with Parmesan.

Makes 4 servings

RAGOUT OF PARSNIPS AND BUTTERNUT SQUASH

Parsnips and squash conspire to form a delectable stewlike dish exuding with the comforting scent of paprika and oregano. Serve this European-style ragout with something green such as steamed broccoli, asparagus, or braised escarole, and a big helping of rice.

1½ tablespoons canola oil
1 medium yellow onion, diced
1 medium red bell pepper, seeded and diced
2 cloves garlic, minced
1 large tomato, diced
1 tablespoon paprika
1 tablespoon dried oregano
½ teaspoon salt
½ teaspoon black pepper
2 cups water
2 cups peeled, diced parsnips
2 cups peeled, diced butternut or buttercup squash

In a medium saucepan, heat the oil. Add the onion, pepper, and garlic and sauté for about 4 minutes. Add the tomato and seasonings and sauté for 5 minutes more. Add the water, parsnips, and squash and cook for about 30 minutes over medium-low heat, stirring occasionally. Remove from the heat and let stand for 10 minutes.

Serve with steamed broccoli or asparagus and a mound of rice.

Makes 4 servings

SPAGHETTI WITH EGGPLANT-TOMATO RAGOUT

I grew up on spaghetti, subsisted on it throughout college, and later, as an adult, vigorously avoided it altogether. Call it Noodle Overload. But time heals most wounds, and I have come to reappreciate this original, pregourmet pasta. This simple yet satisfying dish helped rekindle my enthusiasm for good ol' "spaghet."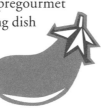

½ pound spaghetti
1½ tablespoons olive oil
1 small yellow onion, diced
1 medium eggplant, diced
1 small summer squash, diced
2 cloves garlic, minced
4 large tomatoes, diced
2 teaspoons dried oregano
2 teaspoons dried basil
½ teaspoon salt
¼ teaspoon red pepper flakes
2 ounces grated Parmesan cheese or shredded part-skim mozzarella

In a medium saucepan, place the spaghetti in enough boiling water to cover, stir, and return to a boil. Cook according to package directions (for al dente, about 9 to 11 minutes). Drain in a colander and keep warm.

Meanwhile, in a medium saucepan, heat the oil. Add the onion, eggplant, squash, and garlic and sauté for 5 to 7 minutes. Add the tomatoes and seasonings and cook for 15 minutes more over medium heat, stirring frequently.

Place the spaghetti on serving plates and ladle the ragout over the top. Sprinkle with Parmesan cheese and serve with Italian bread and a bottle of red wine.

Makes 3 to 4 servings

CURRIED EGGPLANT AND POTATO STEW

Called *aloo beingan*, this savory, easy-to-prepare meal of potatoes, eggplant, and chickpeas is an Indian delight. I have found that the best curry dishes are directly correlated to the quality of the curry powder. It pays to use a premium curry from either India or the West Indies.

1½ tablespoons canola oil
1 medium yellow onion, diced
1 medium green bell pepper, seeded and diced
1 tablespoon minced gingerroot
2 medium tomatoes, diced
2 cups diced eggplant
2 to 3 teaspoons curry powder
1 tablespoon dried parsley
½ teaspoon salt
¼ teaspoon ground cloves
¼ teaspoon cayenne pepper
¼ teaspoon ground fenugreek (optional)
2 cups unpeeled, diced white potatoes
2 cups water
1 15-ounce can chickpeas, drained

In a large saucepan, heat the oil. Add the onion, pepper, and gingerroot and sauté over medium heat for 5 minutes. Add the tomatoes and eggplant and cook for 4 minutes more over medium heat, stirring frequently. Add the seasonings and cook for 1 minute more.

Stir in the potatoes and water and cook for about 30 minutes over medium-low heat, stirring occasionally, until the potatoes are tender. Stir in the chickpeas and cook for 5 to 10 minutes more. Serve with basmati rice and plain low-fat yogurt.

Makes 4 servings

KITCHEN TIPS
• Fenugreek is available in natural food stores and Indian specialty markets.

SPICY SQUASH AND CHICKPEA CURRY

Butternut squash is as versatile and easy to pre-pare as a potato, and sometimes even poses as one. Here the winter gourd is spiced with gingerroot and garlic, giving this recipe the culinary rhythm and melody of curry dishes.

1½ tablespoons canola oil
4 cups peeled, chopped butternut squash
2 medium yellow onions, diced
2 medium-size ripe tomatoes, diced
3 to 4 cloves garlic, minced
1 jalapeño or cayenne pepper, seeded and
  minced
1 tablespoon minced gingerroot
1½ tablespoons curry powder
2 teaspoons ground cumin
½ teaspoon black pepper
½ teaspoon salt
¼ teaspoon ground cloves
2 cups water
1 15-ounce can chickpeas, drained

In a large saucepan, heat the oil. Add the squash and onions and cook over medium heat for 4 minutes, stirring occasionally. Add the toma-toes, garlic, pepper, and gingerroot and cook for 4 minutes more. Add the seasonings and cook for 1 minute more, stirring frequently. Stir in the water and cook for 30 to 35 minutes, until the squash is tender. Stir in the chickpeas and cook for 5 to 10 minutes more over low heat.

Remove from the heat and serve over basmati or jasmine rice.

Makes 6 servings

KITCHEN TIPS
- Other winter squash, such as buttercup and Hubbard, can also be used.

VEGETABLE QUINOA BAKE

Quinoa, the ancient South American grain with a nutty flavor and chewy texture, teams up with a medley of vegetables for this casserole-style dish. This makes an impressive centerpiece for holiday dinners or other festive occasions. I prepared this dish on "Alive and Wellness," a cable television show, and it was a big hit.

  1 tablespoon canola oil
  1 medium yellow onion, chopped
  8 to 10 medium button mushrooms, sliced
  1 large green or red bell pepper, seeded and diced
  1 jalapeño pepper, seeded and minced (optional)
  1 small zucchini, diced
  2 cloves garlic, minced
  3 cups water
  1½ cups quinoa, rinsed and drained
  2 cups peeled, diced butternut squash or red kuri squash
  1 cup peeled, diced carrots
  1 cup chopped kale, spinach, or escarole
  1½ tablespoons dried parsley
  ½ teaspoon salt
  ½ teaspoon black pepper

Preheat the oven to 400°F.

In a large saucepan, heat the oil. Add the onion, mushrooms, bell pepper, jalapeño pepper, if desired, zucchini, and garlic and sauté for about 5 to 7 minutes. Stir in the water, quinoa, squash, carrots, kale, and seasonings and bring to a boil.

Transfer the mixture to a 9″ × 13″ casserole dish and cover. Bake for 30 to 40 minutes, until all of the liquid is absorbed.

Remove from the oven and fluff with a fork. Let stand for 5 minutes before serving.

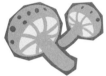

Makes 6 to 8 servings

CARIBE VEGETABLE SANCOCHO

Sancocho is a stew of tropical root vegetables, plantains, and pumpkin. It is the pot-au-feu of the Caribbean. The exotic ingredients (yuca, dasheen, and plantains) can be found in Caribbean and Hispanic markets or in the specialty produce sections of well-stocked grocery stores.

1½ tablespoons canola oil
1 medium yellow onion, diced
1 medium green bell pepper, seeded and diced
2 cloves garlic, minced
4 cups water
2 medium carrots, peeled and diced
2 cups peeled, diced yuca or dasheen
1 cup peeled, diced white potatoes
1 cup peeled, diced West Indian pumpkin or butternut squash
1 medium yellow plantain, peeled and sliced thick
6 whole cloves
2 tablespoons dried parsley
1 tablespoon dried oregano
2 teaspoons dried thyme leaves
½ teaspoon black pepper
½ teaspoon salt

In a large saucepan, heat the oil. Add the onion, bell pepper, and garlic and sauté for about 7 minutes. Add the water, carrots, yuca, potatoes, pumpkin, plantain, and seasonings. Cook over medium-low heat for 40 to 45 minutes, stirring occasionally, until the vegetables are tender and stewlike. Remove from the heat and let stand for 10 minutes.

Serve with Bayou Red Beans and Caribbean Heat Salad or Lemon-Braised Autumn Greens (see Index for recipes).

Makes 6 servings

INDONESIAN FRIED RICE (NASI GORENG)

In Indonesia, fried rice (called nasi goreng) is eaten anytime of day or night. The rice is flavored with ketjap manis, a sweetened version of soy sauce. (I pour ketjap manis over rice the way one pours ketchup over French fries.) The addition of chopped cucumbers offers a cooling contrast to the chili-spiced rice.

1 tablespoon canola oil
1 medium yellow onion, chopped fine
8 medium button mushrooms, sliced
4 shallots, minced
1 to 2 hot red chili peppers, seeded and minced (optional)
2 medium tomatoes, diced
1 teaspoon paprika
4 cups cooked long-grain rice, preferably basmati
8 broccoli florets, blanched
1 to 2 tablespoons ketjap manis (or light soy sauce mixed with 1 teaspoon brown sugar)
1 medium cucumber, peeled and chopped fine

In a large skillet, heat the oil. Add the onion, mushrooms, shallots, and chilies, if desired, and sauté for about 3 minutes. Add the tomatoes and paprika and sauté for 4 minutes more, until the vegetables are tender. Stir in the rice, broccoli, and ketjap manis and cook over medium heat, stirring continuously, until the rice is steaming.

Spoon the fried rice onto serving plates and top with the cucumber. Pass the bottle of ketjap manis at the table.

Makes 4 servings

KITCHEN TIPS

• Ketjap manis is available in Asian specialty stores and in the Asian section of well-stocked grocery stores.

WEST AFRICAN JOLLOF RICE

This meatless adaptation of a traditional West African "party dish" makes a colorful and high-spirited main course.

1 tablespoon vegetable oil
1 medium yellow onion, chopped fine
1 medium green bell pepper, seeded and diced
1 tablespoon minced gingerroot
1 jalapeño pepper, seeded and minced (optional)
2 medium tomatoes, diced
2 to 3 teaspoons curry powder
2 teaspoons dried thyme leaves
½ teaspoon black pepper
½ teaspoon salt
1½ cups long-grain white rice
3 cups water or vegetable stock
2 large carrots, peeled and diced
1 tablespoon tomato paste
2 cups chopped leafy green vegetables (spinach, kale, or chard)
1 15-ounce can black-eyed peas or pigeon peas, drained

In a large saucepan, heat the oil. Add the onion, bell pepper, gingerroot, and jalapeño, if desired, and sauté for about 7 minutes. Add the tomatoes and seasonings and sauté for 1 to 2 minutes more. Stir in the rice, water or stock, carrots, and tomato paste. Cover and cook over medium-low heat for about 15 minutes.

Stir in the spinach (or other greens) and peas and cook for about 5 minutes more over low heat. Fluff the rice and let stand for 10 minutes before serving. Serve with Oven-Roasted Sweet Plantains (see Index).

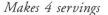

Makes 4 servings

MIDDLE EASTERN LENTIL AND BULGUR STEW

When I'm in the mood for something nourishing and different that doesn't require a lot of time or ingredients, I make this dish. It's another one of my grandmother's specialties—she calls it *imjadara*.

> *1 cup dried green lentils, rinsed*
> *4½ cups water*
> *½ cup coarse bulgur (cracked wheat)*
> *½ teaspoon salt*
> *½ teaspoon black pepper*
> *1 to 2 tablespoons olive oil*
> *1 medium yellow onion, slivered*

In a medium saucepan, combine the lentils and water and bring to a simmer over medium heat. Cook for about 25 minutes; then add the bulgur, salt, and pepper. Cook for 15 to 20 minutes more, stirring frequently, until the lentils are tender. Add a little hot water if necessary.

In a small skillet, heat the oil. Add the onion and sauté for 7 to 10 minutes, until browned. Stir the onion into the pot of lentils and bulgur. Serve hot with pita bread and Emily's Spinach and Shredded Beet Salad (see Index) or a tossed green salad.

Makes 3 to 4 servings

LEMONY BULGUR PILAF

Bulgur pilaf is enjoyed in most Eastern Mediterranean countries. For the best results, use coarse bulgur for this recipe, as opposed to the fine bulgur found in tabouleh. A touch of fresh lemon lightly coats the grains with a pleasant citrusy nuance.

> *1½ cups coarse bulgur (cracked wheat)*
> *3 cups water*
> *3 tablespoons minced fresh parsley (or 1½ tablespoons dried)*
> *1 teaspoon ground cumin*
> *1 teaspoon ground coriander*
> *½ teaspoon black pepper*
> *½ teaspoon salt*
> *1½ tablespoons olive oil*
> *1 medium yellow onion, chopped fine*
> *1 medium green or red bell pepper, seeded and slivered*
> *1 medium yellow zucchini or patty pan squash, slivered*
> *2 scallions, chopped*
> *1 lemon, quartered*

In a medium saucepan, combine the bulgur, water, and seasonings, cover, and bring to a boil. Turn off the heat and let stand for 15 minutes, or until the bulgur has absorbed all of the water.

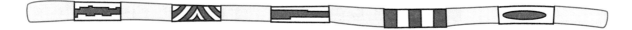

In another medium saucepan, heat the oil. Add the onion, pepper, and squash and sauté for about 7 minutes. Stir in the bulgur and scallions and cook for a few minutes more over medium heat.

Squeeze the lemon over the pilaf; serve hot.

Makes 4 servings

DUTCH SPLIT PEA AND BARLEY STEW

This wholesome creation was inspired by the split pea stews for which Holland is known. When it's in season, I like to add a root vegetable, such as parsnip or small rutabaga, in place of the potato. Other grains, such as quinoa or brown rice, may be used in place of barley.

1½ tablespoons olive oil
1 medium yellow onion, diced
1 cup sliced celery
2 large carrots, peeled and diced
3 to 4 cloves garlic, minced
6 cups water
1 cup dried green split peas, rinsed
½ cup pearl barley

2 large white potatoes or yams, peeled and chopped coarse
2 tablespoons dried parsley
2 teaspoons dried oregano or thyme leaves
½ teaspoon black pepper
2 cups chopped escarole, chard, or spinach
About 1 teaspoon salt

In a large saucepan, heat the oil. Add the onion, celery, carrots, and garlic and sauté for about 7 minutes. Add the water, split peas, barley, potatoes, and seasonings, except the salt, and bring to a simmer. Cook over medium heat for about 1 hour, stirring occasionally, until the peas are tender. Stir in the escarole and cook over low heat for 10 minutes more.

Spoon the stew into shallow serving plates and add salt to taste. Serve with a hunk of European style bread.

Makes 6 servings

KITCHEN TIPS
• To expedite the cooking time, soak the split peas a few hours before cooking. Discard the soaking liquid.

CHILEAN PUMPKIN, CORN, AND BEAN STEW

Pumpkin, corn, and beans (known as "the three sisters" because of the way they grow together) were life-sustaining crops in the pre-Columbian Americas. In Chile, they inspired this harvest stew known as *porotos granados*, or "grand beans." For the full-blown treatment, present it in a Baked Pumpkin (see Index).

1½ tablespoons canola oil
1 medium yellow onion, diced
2 to 3 cloves garlic, minced
1 jalapeño pepper, seeded and minced
2 large tomatoes, diced
1 tablespoon paprika
1 tablespoon dried oregano
1 tablespoon dried parsley
1 teaspoon ground cumin
½ teaspoon salt
4 cups peeled, diced pumpkin, red kuri, or
  butternut squash
2 cups water
2 cups corn kernels, fresh or frozen and
  thawed
1 15-ounce can cranberry beans or red
  kidney beans, drained

In a large saucepan, heat the oil. Add the onion, garlic, and chili pepper and sauté for about 5 minutes. Add the tomatoes and seasonings and cook for about 3 to 4 minutes more, stirring frequently. Add the pumpkin and water and cook for about 30 minutes, stirring occasionally, until the pumpkin is tender. Stir in the corn and beans and cook for about 10 minutes more over low heat. To thicken, mash the pumpkin against the side of the pan.

Serve over a bed of quinoa, brown rice, or couscous.

Makes 4 servings

SOUTH AMERICAN VEGETABLE STEW

This rustic dish, called *locro* in some South American countries, is a rustic stew that is often served with rice. For the meatless version, a South American squash called *zapallo* is used (butternut squash or West Indian pumpkin are similar). My friend, Jessica Robin, who traveled extensively throughout Bolivia, Chile, and Peru, was a consultant on this recipe.

1 tablespoon canola oil

1 medium yellow onion, diced

2 to 3 cloves garlic, minced

1 jalapeño or Red Fresno pepper, seeded and minced (optional)

3 to 4 large tomatoes, diced

2 tablespoons dried parsley

1 tablespoon paprika

1 tablespoon dried oregano

½ teaspoon salt

½ teaspoon black pepper

4 cups peeled, diced zapallo, West Indian pumpkin, buttercup, or butternut squash

3 cups water

2 cups corn kernels, fresh or frozen

4 to 6 cups cooked brown or white rice

In a large saucepan, heat the oil. Add the onion, garlic, and chili pepper, if desired, and sauté for about 5 minutes. Add the tomatoes and seasonings and cook for 4 to 5 minutes more, until the mixture forms a thick pulp. Add the squash and water (and corn, if fresh off the cob) and cook for 25 to 30 minutes over medium heat, stirring occasionally, until the squash is tender. Add the corn (if frozen) and cook for about 10 minutes more over low heat.

To thicken the stew, mash the squash against the side of the pan with the back of a spoon. Serve with plenty of rice and braised leafy greens.

Makes 4 to 6 servings

KITCHEN TIPS
- Zapallo and West Indian pumpkin are available in many Caribbean and Latin American markets.

BRAZILIAN FEIJOADA

Feijoada, the national dish of Brazil, is a bois-terous black bean stew brimming with robust flavors (*feijao* means beans in Portuguese). The dish is served everywhere in Brazil, from beach-side stands to the finest restaurants. This ver-sion captures the spirit of feijoada minus the meat. Chipotle pepper adds a veneer of smoky heat.

1½ cups dried black beans, soaked overnight and drained
1 tablespoon canola oil
1 large yellow onion, diced
2 medium red or green bell peppers, seeded and diced
1 large tomato, diced
4 cloves garlic, minced
1 to 2 canned chipotle peppers, chopped
2 cups peeled, diced sweet potatoes, butternut squash, or white potatoes
2 teaspoons dried thyme leaves
¼ cup chopped fresh parsley (or 2 tablespoons dried)
1 teaspoon salt
4 to 6 cups cooked white or brown rice

In a medium saucepan, place the beans in plenty of water and cook for about 1 hour, over medium heat, until tender. Drain and reserve 2 cups of the cooking liquid.

In a large saucepan, heat the oil. Add the onion, bell peppers, tomato, garlic, and chipo-tle peppers and sauté for 8 to 10 minutes. Add the beans, cooking liquid, sweet potatoes, and thyme and cook for 25 to 30 minutes over medium heat, stirring occasionally. Stir in the parsley and salt and cook for 5 to 10 minutes more.

Spoon the rice into bowls and ladle the fei-joada over the top. Serve with Garlic Braised Rapini (see Index) or steamed spinach.

Makes 6 servings

KITCHEN TIPS
- Chipotle peppers are sold in the Mexican specialty section of well-stocked grocery stores.

SWEET POTATO AND BROCCOLI SAMBAR

Sambar is a Sri Lankan curry dish consisting of lentils, vegetables, and potatoes. One key seasoning is fenugreek, a fragrant spice that adds a deep resonance to curry dishes. Sambar is typically served with Mint Leaf–Coconut Chutney (see Index) on the side.

> *1 cup green or red lentils, rinsed*
> *5 cups water*
> *1 tablespoon canola oil*
> *1 medium yellow onion, diced*
> *2 cloves garlic, minced*
> *1 large tomato, diced*
> *2 teaspoons Madras or other quality curry powder*
> *½ teaspoon ground fenugreek*
> *½ teaspoon ground coriander*
> *½ teaspoon salt*
> *¼ teaspoon cayenne pepper*
> *¼ teaspoon turmeric*
> *2 medium carrots, peeled and diced*
> *1 large sweet potato, scrubbed and diced*
> *10 to 12 small broccoli florets*

In a medium saucepan, place the lentils and water and cook for about 45 minutes, until tender. Drain and reserve about 2 cups of the cooking liquid.

In a large skillet, heat the oil. Add the onion and garlic and sauté for 3 minutes. Add the tomato, reduce the heat, and cook for 3 minutes more, stirring frequently. Stir in the seasonings and cook for 1 minute more, stirring frequently. Add the carrots, potato, lentils, and 1½ cups of the cooking liquid and cook for 20 to 30 minutes over medium-low heat, stirring occasionally. If the curry is too thick, add more liquid.

Stir in the broccoli and let stand for 10 minutes off of the heat. Serve the sambar over basmati or jasmine rice. Mint Leaf–Coconut Chutney or Cucumber Cool Down (see Index for recipes) make natural accompaniments.

Makes 4 servings

KITCHEN TIPS

- Fenugreek is available in the spice sections of natural food stores and Indian specialty markets.

ROOT VEGETABLE AND SQUASH AU GRATIN

There's something intrinsically comforting about the sight of hardy vegetables roasting in the pan. This homestyle casserole can be made with nondairy soy milk instead of cow's milk, if desired.

> *1 tablespoon canola oil*
> *1 small yellow onion, diced*
> *2 cups diced zucchini*
> *2 cloves garlic, minced*
> *1½ cups milk or soy milk*
> *4 scallions, chopped*
> *1 tablespoon dried basil*
> *2 teaspoons dried thyme leaves*
> *½ teaspoon black pepper*
> *½ teaspoon salt*
> *2 cups peeled, diced butternut squash*
> *2 cups peeled, diced parsnips or rutabaga*
> *¼ pound green beans, cut into 1-inch sections*
> *¼ cup bread crumbs*
> *About 1 cup shredded Gruyère cheese (optional)*

Preheat the oven to 375°F.

In a medium saucepan, heat the oil. Add the onion, zucchini, and garlic and sauté for 7 minutes. Add the milk, scallions, and seasonings and bring to a simmer. Remove from the heat.

Layer the butternut squash, parsnips, and green beans in the bottom of a 9″ × 13″ casserole or gratin dish. Pour the vegetable-milk mixture over the top. Sprinkle the bread crumbs and, if desired, the cheese over the top. Place in the oven and bake for 30 to 35 minutes, until a crust forms and the vegetables are tender.

Remove from the oven and let stand for 10 minutes before serving.

Makes 6 servings

ROTI WITH POTATO-CHICKPEA CURRY

Roti is a fat, overflowing skillet-cooked sandwich. The roti ("rowtee") dough is rolled to a thin, elastic consistency, similar to a samosa or tortilla, and stuffed with curried vegetables. It is then cooked on a roti iron or a wide skillet. Roti originated in Trinidad and is served throughout the Caribbean. This adaptation is based on a memorable dish I devoured on the quaint island of St. Thomas.

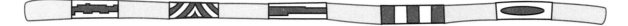

FOR THE ROTI DOUGH:

4 cups unbleached all-purpose flour
2 teaspoons baking powder
1 teaspoon salt
4 tablespoons canola oil
1 cup plus 2 tablespoons water

FOR THE FILLING:

1 tablespoon canola oil
1 small red onion, chopped fine
2 cloves garlic, minced
1 tablespoon curry powder
1 teaspoon ground cumin
½ teaspoon black pepper
½ teaspoon salt
4 cups peeled, diced white potatoes or sweet
*   potatoes*
2 medium carrots, peeled and diced
1½ cups water
1 15-ounce can chickpeas, drained
Vegetable spray

To make the dough, combine the dry ingredients in a large mixing bowl. Gradually add the oil and water to the bowl, mixing and kneading the dough as you go. Form a large ball with an elastic texture. Cover the dough with wax paper and set aside for 30 minutes to 1 hour.

To make the filling, in a medium skillet, heat the oil. Add the onion and garlic and sauté for 4 to 5 minutes. Add the seasonings and cook for 1 minute more over low heat, stirring frequently. Add the potatoes, carrots, and water and cook for 15 to 20 minutes over medium heat, until the potatoes are tender. Stir in the chickpeas and cook for 5 to 10 minutes more, until the filling is chunky and thick. Mash the potatoes against the side of the pan to thicken. Set aside.

Divide the dough into 6 equal balls. On wax paper or a floured surface, flatten each ball and roll out into thin 8-inch rounds or squares. Fill the middle of each with a little more than ½ cup of the filling. Fold the dough over the top of the filling and seal the edges with the back of a fork.

To cook the roti, heat a lightly sprayed, wide skillet or roti iron over medium-high heat. Pick up a filled roti with a large spatula and place in the pan. Cook for 4 to 5 minutes, until the crust is golden brown. Turn with the spatula and continue cooking until golden brown. Repeat the process with the remaining rotis. Serve with bottled hot sauce and tossed greens.

Makes 6 servings

VEGETABLE BARLEY JAMBALAYA

Jambalaya is a rowdy, highly spiced Creole dish. Although usually made with rice, this variation uses pearl barley, which is equally inviting. Traditional jambalaya also contains meat, but a cornucopia of vegetables is infinitely more interesting. This makes a lively party dish.

1 cup pearl barley
3½ cups hot water
1½ tablespoons canola oil
1 medium green bell pepper, seeded and diced
1 small yellow onion, diced
1 small eggplant or zucchini, diced
8 to 10 medium button mushrooms, sliced
1 celery stalk, sliced
2 cloves garlic, minced
1 16-ounce can crushed tomatoes
½ cup water
2 teaspoons dried oregano
1½ teaspoons dried thyme
1 to 3 teaspoons Tabasco or other bottled hot sauce
1 teaspoon ground cumin
½ teaspoon salt
½ teaspoon black pepper
¼ teaspoon cayenne pepper
10 to 12 broccoli florets
1 cup cooked or canned red kidney beans, drained (optional)

In a medium saucepan, place the barley and hot water and cook over medium heat for 35 to 45 minutes, stirring occasionally, until the barley is tender. Set aside.

In a large saucepan, heat the oil. Add the green pepper, onion, eggplant, mushrooms, celery, and garlic and cook over medium heat for about 10 minutes, stirring frequently. Add the crushed tomatoes, water, and seasonings. Cook over medium-low heat for 15 to 20 minutes, stirring occasionally. Reduce the heat to low and fold in the cooked barley, broccoli, and beans, if desired. Cook for 10 to 15 minutes more, stirring frequently. Serve with bread and a tossed salad. Pass the Tabasco at the table.

Makes 4 to 6 servings

KITCHEN TIPS
- Sprinkle shredded low-fat provolone cheese over the top before serving.

PAELLA BOUNTIFUL

Paella comes from a term meaning "frying pan" in the Catalan region of Spain. This meatless version of paella makes an attractive, straight-from-the-hearth centerpiece for a holiday celebration or other special occasion. It is a bountiful display of grains and vegetables.

1½ tablespoons olive oil
2 cups sliced leeks
1 medium zucchini, diced
3 to 4 cloves garlic, minced
4 cups water
1½ cups brown rice
½ cup wild rice
2 large carrots, peeled and diced
1 cup green peas, fresh or frozen
2 cobs of corn, shucked and cut into 1-inch sections
¼ cup minced fresh parsley (or 2 tablespoons dried)
2 teaspoons dried thyme leaves
½ teaspoon turmeric
½ teaspoon black pepper
½ teaspoon salt
12 asparagus spears

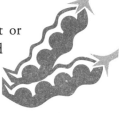

Preheat the oven to 375°F.

In a large cast-iron skillet or Dutch oven, heat the oil. Add the leeks, zucchini, and garlic and cook over medium heat for about 7 minutes, stirring occasionally. Stir in the water, both rices, carrots, peas, corn, and seasonings. Cover and place in the oven and bake for 45 minutes.

Remove the skillet from the oven and fluff the rice. Arrange the asparagus over the top, cover, and bake for 5 to 10 minutes more, until all of the liquid is absorbed. Remove from the heat and let stand for 10 minutes.

Place the skillet on the center of the table and serve hot.

Makes 4 to 6 servings

SUMMER VEGETABLE GRILL WITH CHAMPAGNE VINAIGRETTE

Grilling is one of my favorite pastimes. It imparts a smoky, rustic essence without a lot of namby-pamby fussiness. The champagne vinaigrette in this recipe is perfect for the fun atmosphere that grilling provides.

¼ cup olive oil
¼ cup champagne vinegar
¼ cup chopped mixture of mint, basil, and
    parsley
1 teaspoon brown sugar, packed
2 large tomatoes, halved
1 medium eggplant, cut widthwise into ½-
    inch-thick slices
1 large red onion, peeled and halved
2 medium green or red bell peppers, cut in
    half and seeded
1 medium zucchini, cut widthwise into ½-
    inch-thick slices
10 to 12 medium whole button mushrooms
    or 2 large portobello mushrooms, sliced
Salt and black pepper, to taste

First, make the vinaigrette: In a small bowl, whisk together the oil, vinegar, herbs, and sugar. Set aside for about 30 minutes. (This can be made a day in advance.)

Preheat the grill until the coals are gray to white.

When the fire is ready, place the vegetables on the grill. Cook each side for about 5 to 7 minutes. When the tomatoes are ready to burst, pull them off. Pull the other vegetables off as they become tender.

Coarsely chop the eggplant, red onion, and bell peppers, discarding any charred parts. Add all of the vegetables to the vinaigrette and toss thoroughly. Season with salt and pepper to taste. Serve with couscous, brown rice, or pasta.

Makes 4 servings

JAMAICAN JERK VEGETABLES

In the pantheon of the world's great ethnic dishes, Jamaica's jerk barbecue ranks as one of the greatest. It is sweet, fragrant, hot, spicy, and full of complex flavors. Although originally a meat dish, jerk is easily adapted to the vegetarian grill.

FOR THE VEGETABLES:

1 medium zucchini, chopped coarse
8 cherry tomatoes, halved
1 medium green pepper, seeded and chopped
* coarse*
8 to 10 medium button mushrooms
8 to 10 broccoli florets

FOR THE MARINADE:

6 to 8 scallions, chopped
1 medium yellow onion, diced
½ to 2 Scotch bonnet or jalapeño peppers,
* seeded and minced*
¾ cup light soy sauce
½ cup red wine vinegar
¼ cup canola oil
¼ cup brown sugar, packed
1½ tablespoons fresh thyme (1½ teaspoons
* dried)*

½ teaspoon ground cloves
½ teaspoon nutmeg
½ teaspoon allspice or cinnamon

Thread the vegetables onto 4 barbecue skewers, alternating zucchini, cherry tomato, green pepper, mushroom, and broccoli. Place the skewers in a casserole dish.

In a food processor fitted with a steel blade, add the marinade ingredients. Process for 10 to 15 seconds at high speed. Pour the marinade over the skewered vegetables and refrigerate for 2 to 4 hours.

Preheat the grill until the coals are gray to white.

Remove the skewers from the marinade and drain off any excess liquid. Place on the oiled grill and cook for 4 to 5 minutes on each side, or until the vegetables are tender (not burnt!). Serve with Oven-Roasted Sweet Plantains and Pumpkin Rice and Beans (see Index for recipes) or another rice dish.

Makes 4 servings

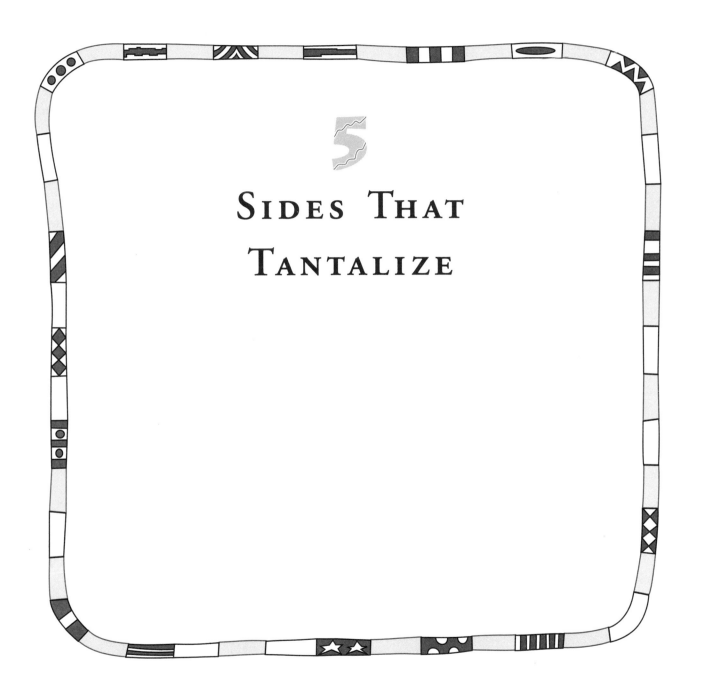

5

SIDES THAT
TANTALIZE

Side dishes have always been meatless territory, the traditional domain of vegetables and starches. Too often, however, the temptation has been to overload a baked potato with sour cream or drown a vegetable in a pool of butter. Here the challenge is to break the routine and prepare side dishes that are high in flavor and low in fat, cholesterol, and salt—and in so doing, move the side dish portion from the "outer edge" to the "cutting edge."

While the side dish plays the supporting role, almost never the lead, it is still an integral part of the meal. It can complement, juxtapose, or provide aesthetic contrast to the main entree. The side dish can even appear in the center of the plate, albeit as a bed for the main dish. Whether on the perimeter or as a prop, the side dish can imbue an ordinary meal with extraordinary flavors.

This chapter offers an ample collection of imaginative recipes, including Pumpkin Rice and Beans, Festive Yellow Rice, Lemon-Braised Autumn Greens, Stove Top Quinoa Pilaf, Black Bean–Jalapeño Succotash, and Oven-Roasted Sweet Plantains. The usual suspects—braised greens, stewed beans, roasted tubers, root vegetables, winter squash, and glorious grains—turn up with renewed vigor.

PUMPKIN RICE AND BEANS

This dish is prepared with West Indian pumpkin, a huge squash enjoyed year-round in the Caribbean. It has a vibrant, sweet, potatolike flesh and melds smoothly with rice for this island version of rice and beans.

1½ tablespoons canola oil

1 medium yellow onion, chopped

2 cloves garlic, minced

2 cups peeled, diced West Indian pumpkin
   or other winter squash

2½ teaspoons curry powder

½ teaspoon black pepper

½ teaspoon salt

¼ teaspoon ground cloves

3 cups water

1½ cups white rice

1 cup coarsely chopped, packed kale or
   spinach

1 15-ounce can red kidney beans or pigeon
   peas, drained

In a large saucepan, heat the oil. Add the onion and garlic and sauté for 5 to 7 minutes, until the onion is soft. Stir in the pumpkin and seasonings and cook for 1 minute more.

Add the water and rice, cover, and cook over medium-low heat for about 15 minutes. Stir in the kale and beans and cook for about 5 min-

utes more. Fluff the rice and turn off the heat. Let stand for 10 to 15 minutes before serving.

Makes 4 to 6 servings

KITCHEN TIPS

- West Indian pumpkin, also called calabaza, is available in many Caribbean and Latin American markets. Hubbard, butternut, or sugar pie pumpkin may be substituted.
- For a taste of island heat, add a whole Scotch bonnet pepper (pierced once with a fork) to the rice while it simmers. Remove it before serving and cut into thin strips, discarding the seeds; serve on the side.

JAMAICAN COOK-UP RICE

Cook-up rice is an island way to use leftover vegetables and rice. "Whatever you have in the kitchen goes into the pot," says Claire Terrelonge, a Jamaican friend of mine. "Think of it as tropical fried rice." A hint of coconut milk endows the dish with a taste of the Caribbean.

1 tablespoon canola oil
1 medium yellow onion, diced
1 medium green bell pepper, seeded and diced
1 medium zucchini or eggplant, diced
8 to 10 medium button mushrooms, sliced
½ to 1 Scotch bonnet pepper or other hot pepper, seeded and minced (optional)
2 cups water
1 cup reduced-fat coconut milk (or water, for a light version)
1½ cups white rice
2 cups peeled, diced winter squash, sweet potato, or carrots
2 tablespoons dried parsley
1 teaspoon dried thyme
½ teaspoon allspice
½ teaspoon salt
2 cups chopped greens (kale, Swiss chard, beet greens, or spinach)
1 15-ounce can red kidney beans or pigeon peas, drained

In a large saucepan, heat the oil. Add the onion, bell pepper, zucchini, mushrooms, and chili pepper, if desired, and sauté for about 7 minutes. Add the water, coconut milk, rice, winter squash, and seasonings. Cover and cook over medium-low heat for 15 to 20 minutes.

Stir in the greens and beans and cook for a few minutes more. Turn off the heat, fluff the rice, and let sit on the stove top for about 10 minutes.

Makes 4 to 6 servings

CURRIED TURNIPS AND SWEET POTATOES

The turnip is a misunderstood and much-maligned root vegetable. When given the chance, however, and paired with the right ingredients, the bulbous root can surprise and reward the patient palate. This Indian preparation is an appetizing example.

1½ tablespoons canola oil
1 medium yellow onion, diced
2 cloves garlic, minced
1 tablespoon minced gingerroot
2 large ripe tomatoes, peeled and diced
1 tablespoon curry powder
1 teaspoon ground cumin
1 teaspoon ground coriander
½ teaspoon salt
¼ teaspoon cayenne pepper
2 cups peeled, diced turnips
2 cups peeled, diced sweet potatoes
2 cups water
1 15-ounce can chickpeas, drained
  (optional)

In a large saucepan, heat the oil. Add the onion, garlic, and gingerroot and sauté for about 4 minutes. Add the tomatoes and sauté for 4 minutes more. Add the seasonings and cook for 1 minute more over low heat, stirring frequently.

Stir in the turnips, potatoes, and water and cook for 35 to 40 minutes over medium heat, stirring occasionally, until the turnips and potatoes are tender. Stir in the chickpeas, if desired, and cook for 5 to 10 minutes more over low heat.

Serve with basmati or jasmine rice on the side.

Makes 4 servings

ROASTED ROOT VEGETABLES SCENTED WITH THYME

Americans are just recently developing an interest in rutabagas, turnips, and parsnips. Roasting the vegetables is an optimal way to nurture their undiluted flavors.

> *1 large sweet potato, chopped coarse*
> *1 large rutabaga, peeled and diced*
> *1 large parsnip, peeled and diced*
> *2 medium turnips, diced*
> *6 to 8 whole cloves garlic, peeled*
> *3 to 4 tablespoons canola oil*
> *1 tablespoon dried thyme leaves*
> *½ teaspoon salt*
> *½ teaspoon black pepper*
> *1 small bunch thyme sprigs*

Preheat the oven to 375°F.

In a medium mixing bowl, toss together the root vegetables, garlic, oil, spices, and half of the thyme sprigs. Place the vegetables in a casserole dish or baking pan and roast for about 1 hour, until the vegetables are tender. Stir the vegetables every 20 minutes or so.

Remove the vegetables from the oven and let cool slightly before serving. Place the vegetables on a platter and arrange the remaining thyme sprigs around the edges.

Makes 6 servings

KITCHEN TIPS

• If you are without a sweet potato, a rutabaga, a parsnip, or a turnip, you may substitute other roots such as beets, carrots, Jerusalem artichokes, or Caribbean yams, or you may add whole mushrooms or baby onions to the mix instead.

• For a light finish, drizzle a little balsamic vinegar over the platter of vegetables just before serving.

BLACK-EYED PEAS WITH SPINACH AND BULGUR

This Middle Eastern equivalent of rice and beans is a seamless blending of grains, legumes, and greens. It emanates with nutrients and comforting aromas. Crispy brown onions, added at the finish, really make the dish.

> *2½ cups water*
> *3 to 4 cups chopped fresh spinach*
> *1 15-ounce can black-eyed peas, drained*
> *1 cup coarse grain bulgur (cracked wheat)*
> *½ teaspoon salt*
> *½ teaspoon black pepper*
> *1 to 1½ tablespoons canola oil or olive oil*
> *2 medium yellow onions, sliced thin*

In a large saucepan, bring the water to a boil. Add the spinach and black-eyed peas and cook for about 5 minutes over medium heat. Stir in the bulgur and seasonings. Remove from the heat, cover, and let stand for about 15 minutes.

In a small skillet, heat the oil. Add the onions and sauté for 7 to 10 minutes, until golden brown. Set aside.

Drain any excess water from the bulgur mixture and spoon into serving bowls. Cover with the sautéed onions and serve at once.

Makes 4 servings

OVEN-ROASTED SWEET PLANTAINS

Plantains are a popular starch in African, Caribbean, and Hispanic kitchens. They resemble wild, prehistoric-looking bananas. Unlike bananas, however, plantains must be cooked to be eaten. Green plantains ripen to yellow and develop black patches. This is okay. Despite their spotted appearance, ripe plantains are at their most desirable level—sweet, tender, and bananalike.

Plantains are often fried, but roasting them is a healthful alternative.

2 to 3 large ripe plantains
¼ teaspoon nutmeg, allspice, or cinnamon

Preheat the oven to 400°F.

Cut off the tips of the plantains. Place the plantains on a baking sheet and bake for 15 to 20 minutes, until the skin is charred and puffy.

Take the plantains out of the oven and let cool for a few minutes. Slice the plantains down the center lengthwise and peel back the skin. Cut the plantains in half widthwise, sprinkle with nutmeg, and transfer to serving plates.

Makes 4 servings

KITCHEN TIPS
- To ripen green plantains, set them out at room temperature for 5 to 7 days. Storing them in a paper bag will expedite the process. (Do not refrigerate.)

FESTIVE YELLOW RICE

This fragrant dish (called *nasi kuning*) is served at Indonesian weddings, birthdays, and other gala occasions. It is usually mounded in the center of the plate and surrounded with exotic regional delicacies.

> 1 tablespoon canola oil
> 2 tablespoons minced shallots or red onion
> 2 teaspoons minced gingerroot
> 2 teaspoons minced lemon grass
> 1 small jalapeño pepper, seeded and minced
> 1 teaspoon coriander
> ½ teaspoon turmeric
> ½ teaspoon salt
> ⅓ cup currants or dark raisins
> 1 cup long-grain white rice
> 2 cups water

In a medium saucepan, heat the oil. Add the shallots, gingerroot, lemon grass, and chili and sauté for 3 minutes. Add the seasonings and cook for 1 minute more. Stir in the currants, rice, and water and bring to a simmer over medium heat. Cover the pan and cook for 15 to 20 minutes, until the rice is tender.

Remove from the heat, fluff the rice, and keep warm until ready to serve.

Makes 4 servings

DANDELION RICE WITH SWEET POTATOES

Tired of the same old rice dish? It may be time to reinvigorate your rice repertoire. Dandelion greens (a Southern leafy vegetable) and sweet potatoes jazz things up a bit. Although any rice will do, basmati is one of my favorites for this dish.

> 1 medium sweet potato, scrubbed and diced
> 1 large tomato, chopped
> 3 cups water
> 1½ cups long-grain white rice or basmati rice
> ½ teaspoon black pepper
> ½ teaspoon salt
> 2 cups chopped dandelion greens or other Southern greens

In a large saucepan, combine the sweet potato, tomato, water, rice, and seasonings and bring to a boil. Cover and cook over medium-low heat for about 12 minutes. Stir in the greens and cook for about 5 minutes more. Fluff the rice and turn off the heat. Let stand for 10 to 15 minutes before serving.

Makes 4 servings

- For a heartier dish, add 1 15-ounce can of red kidney beans or black-eyed peas along with the greens.
- If dandelions are not available, try mustard greens, turnip greens, or mizuna.
- Mizuna is a tasty Japanese leaf that is available in natural food stores and well-stocked supermarkets.

STOVE TOP QUINOA PILAF

If you have never tried quinoa, this is a good dish to "test the waters." Quinoa is a protein-rich grain with a nutty flavor. It cooks up just like rice.

1 tablespoon canola oil
1 small yellow onion, chopped
6 to 8 medium button mushrooms, sliced
1 medium green or red bell pepper, seeded and diced
1 small zucchini, diced
2 cups water
1 cup quinoa, rinsed
1 cup peeled, diced winter squash, sweet potato, or carrot (something orange)

2 tablespoons chopped fresh parsley (or 1 tablespoon dried)
½ teaspoon black pepper
½ to 1 teaspoon salt

In a medium saucepan, heat the oil. Add the onion, mushrooms, pepper, and zucchini and sauté for 5 to 7 minutes, until tender. Add the water, quinoa, squash, and seasonings and cover. Cook over medium-low heat for 15 to 20 minutes, until all the liquid is absorbed. Fluff the quinoa (like rice) and keep warm until ready to serve.

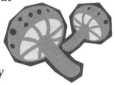

Makes 4 servings

KITCHEN TIPS

- Rinsing the quinoa washes away its natural but unappetizing coating, which has a bitter, soapy flavor. Quinoa is available in natural food stores and in the grains section of well-stocked supermarkets.

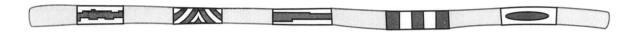

BLACK BEAN–JALAPEÑO SUCCOTASH

The Native American dish of beans and corn is traditionally prepared with lima beans, but black beans and jalapeños make for a tantalizing variation.

> 1 tablespoon canola oil
> 1 small yellow onion, chopped fine
> 1 medium red or green bell pepper, seeded and diced
> 2 cloves garlic, minced
> 1 jalapeño pepper, seeded and minced
> 2 cups corn kernels, fresh or frozen and thawed
> 1 15-ounce can black beans, drained
> 1 teaspoon dried oregano
> ½ teaspoon black pepper
> ½ teaspoon salt
> 2 tablespoons minced cilantro (optional)

In a medium saucepan, heat the oil. Add the onion, bell pepper, garlic, and jalapeño and sauté for 5 minutes. Add the corn, beans, and seasonings and cook for about 5 minutes more over medium heat, stirring occasionally, until the mixture is steaming. Mix in the cilantro, if desired, and serve at once.

Makes 4 servings

BARBECUED CORN-ON-THE-COB RUBBED WITH LIME

There is an art to barbecuing corn-on-the-cob. First, start with the freshest corn possible. Cook the corn until tender, peel back the roasted husks, rub a little lime over the glistening kernels (forget the butter!), and let the feast begin.

> 4 to 6 ears corn (do not shuck)
> A large pot of cold water
> 1 to 2 limes, quartered
> Salt and black pepper, to taste

Soak the corn in the cold water for 30 minutes. Remove from the water and pat dry.

Preheat the grill until the coals are gray to white.

When the fire is ready, place the unshucked corn on the grill. Cook over moderate heat for 20 to 30 minutes, turning every 5 minutes or so. To check for doneness, peek at the corn and check the tenderness of the kernels.

When the corn is done, remove it from the grill and allow it to cool. Shuck off the husks and discard. (You may want to rinse the corn briefly under hot water.) Rub the lime over the corn and season to taste. Eat at once.

Makes 4 servings

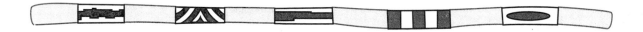

SWEET POTATO SKORDALIA WITH SMOTHERED GREENS

Skordalia is a garlicky sauce rooted in Greek cuisine. Traditionally, it is made with white potatoes and plenty of olive oil. For this lighter version, I've replaced some of the oil with the potato's cooking liquid, and used sweet potatoes just for fun (either potato may be used). Skordalia makes a delectable sauce for braised escarole, spinach, or white beans.

FOR THE SKORDALIA:

> 2 cups peeled, chopped sweet potatoes or
>   white potatoes
> 6 cloves garlic, chopped
> 3 tablespoons olive oil
> 2 teaspoons red wine vinegar
> 2 teaspoons fresh lemon juice
> ¼ teaspoon salt
> ⅛ teaspoon cayenne pepper

FOR THE SMOTHERED GREENS:

> 6 cups chopped escarole, spinach, or rapini
> ¼ cup water
> 8 to 10 leaves arugula

In a small saucepan, place the potatoes in enough boiling water to cover and cook for 15 to 20 minutes, until tender. Drain, reserving about ¼ cup of cooking liquid.

In a food processor fitted with a steel blade, add the garlic and process for about 10 seconds. Add the potatoes, cooking liquid, oil, vinegar, lemon juice, and seasonings and process until smooth. Scrape the skordalia into a serving bowl and keep warm.

In a large saucepan, place the escarole, water, and arugula and cook for 3 to 5 minutes over high heat, until the greens are wilted. Drain the excess liquid and transfer to serving plates. Spoon the skordalia over the top. Pass the extra skordalia at the table. Serve with Tuscan Beans (see Index) and warm bread.

Makes 4 servings

KITCHEN TIPS
- If desired, sprinkle diced walnuts or almonds over the top of the skordalia before serving.
- Arugula is a peppery leafy green available in the produce section of most grocery stores. If unavailable, substitute beet greens or Swiss chard.

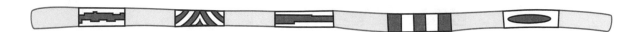

SPICY SQUASH
AND TOMATO CURRY

Squash and curry go together like sugar and spice; they are meant for each other. Although almost any squash will do, my favorite for this dish is the large red kuri, a brilliant reddish-orange squash with a delectable flesh similar to Hubbard squash or West Indian pumpkin. (Red kuri also goes by the name Golden Hubbard.)

    1 tablespoon canola oil
    1 medium red onion, diced
    2 cloves garlic, minced
    1 jalapeño or serrano pepper, seeded and
        minced
    2 to 3 medium-size ripe tomatoes, diced
    2 tablespoons dried parsley
    1 tablespoon curry powder (preferably West
        Indian or Madras)
    1½ teaspoons ground cumin
    ½ teaspoon black pepper
    ½ teaspoon salt
    ¼ teaspoon turmeric
    4 cups peeled, diced red kuri, Hubbard, or
        butternut squash
    2 cups water

In a large saucepan, heat the oil. Add the onion, garlic, and chili pepper and sauté for 4 minutes. Add the tomatoes and sauté for 4 minutes more. Stir in the seasonings and cook for 1 minute more.

Add the squash and water and cook for 30 to 35 minutes over medium heat, stirring occasionally, until the squash is tender. Serve with a main rice dish or other grains.

Makes 4 servings

SOUTHWESTERN GREEN RICE
(ARROZ VERDE)

This staple of the American Southwest and Mexico is a verdant combination of green chilies, spinach, herbs, and rice. Ideally, you would use poblano chilies, which have an eloquent, haunting heat. It is worth the hunt to find them. When they are not available, try substituting a green bell pepper; it's still a rewarding, but milder, dish.

    1½ tablespoons canola oil
    1 medium yellow onion, diced
    2 cloves garlic, minced
    2 roasted poblano chilies or 1 large green
        pepper, seeded and diced
    1 jalapeño pepper, seeded and minced
    2 cups water
    1 cup long-grain white or brown rice

2 tablespoons fresh parsley (or 1 tablespoon dried)
1 teaspoon ground cumin
½ teaspoon salt
¼ teaspoon black pepper
2 cups chopped fresh spinach or other leafy green vegetable
2 tablespoons minced cilantro

In a medium saucepan, heat the oil. Add the onion, garlic, and peppers and sauté for 5 to 7 minutes, until the onions are tender. Add the water, rice, parsley, and dried seasonings and bring to a boil. Cover and cook over medium-low heat for about 15 minutes (for brown rice, about 40 minutes).

Stir in the spinach and cilantro and cook over low heat for about 5 minutes more, until the rice is tender.

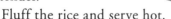

Fluff the rice and serve hot.

Makes 4 servings

KITCHEN TIPS
• Roasting the poblano chilies removes the tough outer skin and produces a smoky flavor (see Index for roasting chilies).

GARLIC-BRAISED RAPINI

Rapini, also called broccoli rabe, is a leafy green vegetable with a hint of mustard and broccoli flavor. It makes a savory side vegetable when prepared in this Italian manner.

2 bunches rapini (about 16 ounces)
2 tablespoons olive oil
2 to 3 cloves garlic, minced
3 to 4 slices stale dark pumpernickel or whole-wheat bread, cubed
Salt and pepper, to taste

Remove and discard the fibrous base stems of the rapini. Rinse the rapini in a colander and pat dry.

In a large, wide skillet, heat the oil. Add the garlic and bread and sauté for 2 to 3 minutes. Stir in the rapini and cook for 3 to 4 minutes more over medium heat, stirring frequently, until the greens are wilted. Transfer to serving plates and season to taste.

Makes 4 servings

KITCHEN TIPS
• Rapini is available in well-stocked supermarkets and Asian markets.

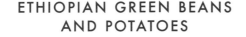

ETHIOPIAN GREEN BEANS AND POTATOES

This wholesome Ethiopian staple (called "yataklete kilkil") is spiced with chilies, turmeric, and lime juice, an exotic blend of enticing flavors.

> *2 large white potatoes, diced (peeled if*
> *desired)*
> *½ pound green beans, cut into 1-inch*
> *sections*
> *1 tablespoon olive oil*
> *1 small yellow onion, chopped fine*
> *2 cloves garlic, minced*
> *1 small jalapeño or serrano pepper, seeded*
> *and minced*
> *½ teaspoon turmeric*
> *½ teaspoon ground cumin*
> *½ teaspoon salt*
> *1 15-ounce can stewed tomatoes*
> *½ teaspoon fresh lime juice*

In a medium saucepan, place the potatoes in enough boiling water to cover and cook for 12 minutes over high heat. Add the green beans and cook for 3 to 5 minutes more. Drain the potatoes and green beans in a colander.

In a large, wide skillet, heat the oil. Add the onion, garlic, and jalapeño and sauté for about 4 minutes. Stir in the seasonings and sauté for 1 minute more. Add the potatoes, green beans, stewed tomatoes, and lime juice and cook for 7 to 10 minutes more over medium heat, stirring frequently.

Transfer to a serving plate and serve at once.

Makes 4 servings

BUTTERMILK MASHED BASIL POTATOES

Buttermilk, despite having the misleading word "butter" in its name, is actually lower in fat than regular milk. It makes a tangy and light replacement for cream in this herb-infused mashed potato recipe.

> *4 cups peeled, diced white potatoes*
> *1 cup buttermilk*
> *¼ cup low-fat milk*
> *½ cup basil or parsley leaves*
> *½ teaspoon salt*
> *¼ teaspoon cayenne pepper*
> *2 scallions, chopped fine*

In a medium saucepan, place the potatoes in enough boiling water to cover and cook for 20 to 25 minutes, until easily pierced with a fork. Drain, discarding the water.

When the potatoes are almost ready, warm the buttermilk and milk in a microwave or in

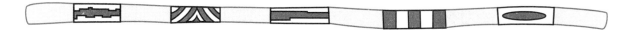

a small saucepan over low heat. (Do not boil.) Transfer the potatoes to a food processor fitted with a steel blade or to a blender and add the buttermilk, milk, basil or parsley, and seasonings. Process until the mixture is smooth. (Leave some chunks for a homemade look.) Transfer to a serving bowl and sprinkle the scallions over the top. Garnish with basil leaves.

Makes 6 servings

ACORN SQUASH WITH SUN-DRIED TOMATO COUSCOUS

Acorn squash, with its pleated, acorn shape and dark green skin, makes a picturesque serving bowl.

1 cup air-packed sun-dried tomatoes
2 medium acorn squash
1 tablespoon canola oil or olive oil
1 small yellow onion, chopped
4 scallions, chopped
2 cloves garlic, minced
1½ cups water
2 tablespoons minced fresh parsley
  (or 1 tablespoon dried)
½ teaspoon black pepper
½ teaspoon salt
1 cup couscous

Soak the tomatoes in warm water for 30 minutes to 1 hour. Drain the liquid and finely chop the tomatoes.

Meanwhile, preheat the oven to 375°F.

Cut the squash in half widthwise and scoop out and discard the seeds and stringy fibers. Place cut-side down on a sheet pan filled with about ¼-inch water. Bake for 35 to 40 minutes, until tender. Remove the squash from the oven, flip over, and let cool for 10 minutes.

In a medium saucepan, heat the oil. Add the onion, scallions, dried tomatoes, and garlic and sauté for about 5 minutes. Stir in the water and seasonings and bring to a boil. Turn off the heat, stir in the couscous, and cover. Let stand for about 10 minutes.

When the squash has cooled, scoop out the flesh, coarsely chop, and blend into the couscous mixture. Fill the hollowed squash with the mixture. Present the stuffed squash on serving platters.

Makes 4 servings

KITCHEN TIPS
- For added body, mix a 15-ounce can of drained chickpeas or red kidney beans into the couscous.

ROASTED SUN CHOKES WITH ROSEMARY

You may know sun chokes by their more common name, Jerusalem artichokes. Oddly enough, Jerusalem artichokes are neither artichokes nor from Jerusalem. The knobby, gingerroot-shaped tubers are native to North America and members of the sunflower family. When sun chokes are roasted like potatoes, they develop a faintly nutty flavor.

> 4 to 6 cloves garlic
> 1½ tablespoons olive oil
> 2 teaspoons dried rosemary (or 1 tablespoon chopped fresh)
> 1½ pounds sun chokes, scrubbed and halved
> About ½ teaspoon paprika
> Salt and black pepper, to taste
> 4 to 8 sprigs rosemary or parsley

Preheat the oven to 400°F.

Combine the garlic, oil, and rosemary in a mixing bowl. Toss in the sun chokes and coat with the mixture. Place the garlic cloves and sun chokes, cut-side down, on a baking pan. Lightly sprinkle paprika over the top and bake for 30 to 40 minutes, until the sun chokes are tender but not mushy.

Transfer to a serving platter and season with salt and pepper to taste. Garnish with sprigs of rosemary or parsley.

Makes 4 servings

BAYOU RED BEANS AND RICE

I discovered the joys of Creole cooking first-hand while I lived in New Orleans years ago. I also learned to appreciate the simple pleasures that a bowl of well-cooked red beans and rice can bring.

> 1 cup red kidney beans, soaked overnight and drained
> 4 cups water
> 1 medium yellow onion, chopped coarse
> 1 medium green bell pepper, diced
> ½ cup sliced celery
> 2 cloves garlic, peeled
> 1 tablespoon dried parsley
> 2 teaspoons dried oregano
> 1 teaspoon dried thyme
> ¼ teaspoon cayenne pepper
> ½ teaspoon salt
> Tabasco or other bottled hot sauce, to taste
> About 4 cups cooked rice

In a medium saucepan, place the beans, water, onion, bell pepper, celery, and garlic and cook for about 1 hour over medium heat, stirring occasionally. Add all of the seasonings (except the salt) and cook for about 30 minutes more, until the beans are tender. Remove the garlic from the pot; discard or give to a garlic lover. Season with salt and Tabasco to taste. Serve over the rice or add to soups or stews.

Makes 4 servings

TUSCAN WHITE BEANS

The region of Tuscany is a haven for bean cuisine. Tuscan-style beans are laden with garlic, sage, and fresh herbs and dressed with a light coating of olive oil. *Mangia!*

> *1 cup white kidney beans (cannellini),*
> *soaked overnight and drained*
> *3½ to 4 cups water*
> *1 small yellow onion, chopped coarse*
> *2 whole cloves garlic*
> *1 teaspoon dried thyme*
> *½ teaspoon sage*
> *½ teaspoon black pepper*
> *2 tablespoons minced parsley or basil*
> *1 to 2 tablespoons olive oil*
> *½ teaspoon salt*

In a medium saucepan, place the beans, water, onion, garlic, thyme, sage, and pepper and cook for about 1 hour over medium heat, stirring occasionally, until the beans are tender. Remove the garlic from the pot; discard or give to a garlic lover. Drain any excess liquid from the beans.

Transfer the beans to a serving bowl and fold in the parsley, oil, and salt. Set aside for 15 minutes to let the flavors intermingle. Serve as a side dish or add to soups or stews.

Makes 4 servings

KITCHEN TIPS
- When in season, blend in 2 to 3 tablespoons of other herbs such as marjoram, oregano, or chives.

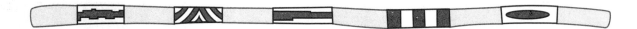

VEGETABLE COUSCOUS

This makes an enticing bed for grilled vegetables, curries, and hearty stews.

1 tablespoon canola oil
1 small yellow onion, diced
1 medium red bell pepper, seeded and diced
1 cup diced zucchini
1 teaspoon paprika
½ teaspoon ground cumin
½ teaspoon salt
½ teaspoon black pepper
1½ cups water
2 scallions, chopped
1 cup couscous
1 15-ounce can red kidney beans or
    chickpeas, drained (optional)

In a medium saucepan, heat the oil. Add the onion, bell pepper, and zucchini and sauté for about 7 minutes. Add the seasonings and cook for 1 minute more. Add the water and scallions and bring to a boil. Stir in the couscous and beans, if desired, cover, and remove from the heat. Let stand for 10 minutes.

Fluff the couscous before serving.

Makes 4 servings

LEMON-BRAISED AUTUMN GREENS

One November past, I went to the farmers' market expecting to find a dwindling supply of winter squash and gourds. What I discovered was a bounty of cascading leafy vegetables of all shapes and shades of green, from emerald to olive. These nutritious cold weather crops invariably put a smiling, optimistic face on autumn and extend the harvest season. A leafy green called red Russian kale is one of my favorites.

1 large bunch Russian kale, field spinach, chard, or Bok choy (about 16 ounces)
1 tablespoon canola or olive oil
1 medium yellow onion, chopped fine
2 cloves garlic, minced
Juice of 1 lemon
½ teaspoon black pepper
½ teaspoon salt
1 tablespoon sesame seeds (optional)

Place the greens in a colander and rinse under cold running water. Remove and discard the stems and coarsely chop the leaves.

In a medium skillet, heat the oil. Add the onion and garlic and sauté for 2 to 3 minutes. Add the greens and lemon juice and cook for about 2 minutes more over low heat, until the greens are wilted. Drain the excess liquid from the pan and place the greens on a shallow serving platter. Season with salt and pepper. Sprinkle the sesame seeds over the top, if desired. Serve as a side to grain or pasta dishes.

Makes 4 servings

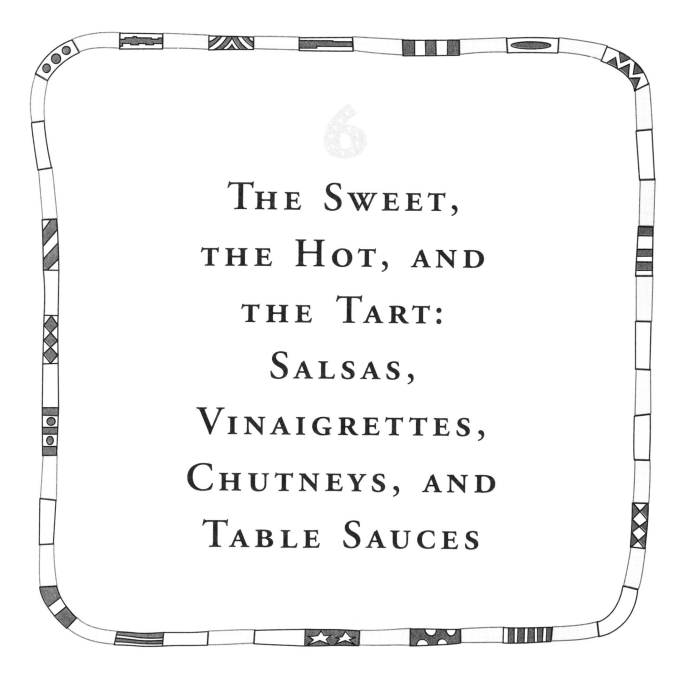

6

THE SWEET,
THE HOT, AND
THE TART:
SALSAS,
VINAIGRETTES,
CHUTNEYS, AND
TABLE SAUCES

To embellish and adorn, heighten and stimulate: this is the credo of a well-made sauce or dressing. Sometimes a meal needs to be perked up, and a spicy salsa or chutney does the trick admirably. Other times, a cool, soothing yogurt accompaniment is welcomed. One thing is assured: there is never a dull meal on the plate with the proper condiment or dressing at the table.

This chapter highlights a new generation of condiments, vinaigrettes, and sauces. From Kiwi Vinaigrette, Cucumber Cool Down, Cranberry Fruit Chutney, and Black Bean Sofrito to Salsa! Salsa! and Arugula-Spinach Pesto, the whole continuum of flavors is covered. These lively, intensely flavored accompaniments have eclipsed the Eurocentric, calorie-laden, fat-drenched sauces

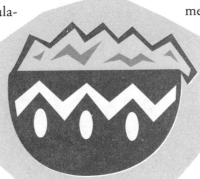

and dressings of the past (hollandaise, bechamel, and the like). Homemade sauces and vinaigrettes are far more delicious and rewarding than many of the sugar-coated, additive-laced commercial counterparts on the market.

Vinegar, low-fat yogurt, and citrus juices have replaced heavy blankets of cream, sour cream, and butter. Fresh fruit purees reinvigorate salad dressings, and mangoes and pineapples contribute a taste of the tropics to sweet-and-tart chutneys. Some table sauces are the slow-cooked pure essence of roasted vegetables and herbs, while other embellishments are whipped up in a matter of minutes. Whether spooned over the top, drizzled from above, or served on the side of a meal, these recipes offer a bonus of pleasing flavors.

KIWI VINAIGRETTE

From the day I offered this clever salad dressing at my restaurant, it became an instant bestseller. It showcases the kiwifruit's versatility. Kiwifruit is much, much more than a fancy garnish for cheesecakes. As an added gift, with fruit in the dressing you don't need nearly as much oil.

4 to 5 ripe kiwifruits, peeled and chopped
  coarse
¼ cup red wine vinegar or apple cider
  vinegar
1 tablespoon honey
½ teaspoon white pepper or black pepper
¼ teaspoon salt
¼ cup plus 1 tablespoon canola oil

In a food processor fitted with a steel blade, place the kiwifruit, vinegar, honey, and seasonings and process for 10 to 15 seconds, until smooth. Slowly drizzle in the oil while the machine is running and process for another 10 seconds. Pour into a serving container and serve at once or refrigerate for later.

Makes about 2 cups (12 to 14 servings)

KITCHEN TIPS

- You can determine the degree of ripeness by holding the kiwi in the palm of your hand and gently pressing down with your thumb; it should give a little.
- For a Papaya-Kiwi Vinaigrette, substitute 1 ripe papaya, peeled and seeded, for 1 or 2 kiwis.

ROASTED EGGPLANT AND SWEET PEPPER RAITA

While Americans prefer sweet yogurt with fruit and sugar (and lately, artificial sugar), cooks in the Middle East and Far East prefer savory yogurt and vegetable combinations. Raita is a soothing Indian yogurt condiment made with a variety of vegetables. Serve with spicy curries.

2 cups plain low-fat yogurt
2 scallions, chopped
2 tablespoons minced cilantro or mint
¼ teaspoon ground cumin
¼ teaspoon coriander
¼ teaspoon cayenne pepper
¼ teaspoon salt
2 medium eggplants, cut in half lengthwise
1 large red bell pepper, halved and seeded

Preheat the broiler.

In a medium mixing bowl, combine the yogurt, scallions, cilantro, and seasonings. Set aside.

Prick the eggplants' skin with a fork. Place the eggplant and pepper cut-side down on a baking pan and, when the broiler is ready, roast the eggplant and pepper beneath the heat until the skin is charred and crackles when touched and the flesh is tender. Remove from the heat and let cool slightly.

Scrape or peel off the charred skin of the eggplant and pepper and discard. Chop the eggplant and blend into the yogurt mixture. Finely chop the pepper and whisk into the yogurt mixture. Serve the raita (warm or cold) as a vegetable dip, sandwich spread, or over a baked potato. It makes a natural accompaniment to almost any curry dish.

Makes 8 servings

KITCHEN TIPS
- If you desire a piquant raita, add 1 to 2 New Mexico chilies or other seasonal chili peppers. For a milder taste, replace the bell pepper with 1 chopped cucumber (skip the roasting, of course).

CUCUMBER COOL DOWN

This is a comforting companion to almost any highly spiced dish. Spoon it over the top or serve it on the side.

2 cups plain low-fat yogurt
1 cup finely chopped cucumber (peeled if desired)
2 tablespoons chopped fresh mint or parsley (or 1 tablespoon dried)

In a small mixing bowl, combine all of the ingredients. Cover and chill until ready to serve.

Makes 6 to 8 servings

KITCHEN TIPS

• Serve with Curried Eggplant and Potato Stew, Red Bean–Quinoa Chili, Sweet Potato and Broccoli Sambar, or New World Borscht (see Index for recipes), or any number of curries or spicy vegetable dishes.

GREEN TOMATO CHUTNEY

Before I became an avid gardener, I never really thought much about green tomatoes. They were tomatoes in waiting, tomatoes to be. But after I picked my first overflowing basketful of green tomatoes (just before the first frost), I learned in a hurry how to cook with them. This sweet-and-tart chutney has become one of my favorite creations.

1 large yellow onion, diced
4 to 5 green tomatoes, diced
4 unpeeled Bartlett pears or apples (any variety except Red Delicious), diced
1 cup red wine vinegar
1 cup apple cider
1 cup dark raisins
½ cup brown sugar, packed
3 to 4 cloves garlic, minced
1 tablespoon minced gingerroot
1 teaspoon ground cumin
½ teaspoon black pepper
½ teaspoon salt
¼ teaspoon ground cloves

In a large, nonreactive saucepan, combine all of the ingredients and cook over medium-low heat for 45 minutes to 1 hour, stirring occasionally, until the mixture is chunky. Remove from the heat and let cool to room temperature; then chill. Reheat and serve with rice, curries, potatoes, or steamed vegetables. If refrigerated, the chutney will keep for several weeks.

Makes 4 cups

SALSA! SALSA!

This is the quintessential tomato salsa: chunky, spicy, complex, radiant with cilantro, lime, and cumin, and, of course, spiked with jalapeño peppers. It's the perfect accompaniment to Jay's Veggie Burrito and Pinto Bean and Corn Quesadilla (see Index for recipes).

2 medium tomatoes, diced
1 medium green bell pepper, seeded and
  diced
1 medium yellow onion, diced
2 cloves garlic, minced
1 to 3 jalapeño peppers, seeded and minced
2 tablespoons chopped cilantro
2 teaspoons fresh lime juice
1 teaspoon ground cumin
1 teaspoon dried oregano
¼ teaspoon black pepper
¼ teaspoon salt
¼ teaspoon cayenne pepper
1 16-ounce can crushed tomatoes

In a large bowl, combine all of the ingredients (except the crushed tomatoes) and mix well. In a food processor fitted with a steel blade, place three-quarters of the mixture and process for 5 to 10 seconds, creating a vegetable mash (not too soupy!).

Return the mash to the bowl and add the crushed tomatoes; blend well. Cover the salsa with plastic wrap and chill for at least 1 hour, allowing the flavors to meld together.

Makes 4 cups

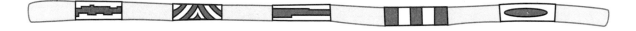

ROASTED VEGETABLE SALSA WITH WATERCRESS

Roasting intensifies the flavors of vegetables, and brings out a rustic quality in this hearty salsa. Watercress has a quiet presence and lends a light herbal touch. This is a good salsa to make in the winter when tomatoes are not quite at their prime.

4 medium tomatoes
1 medium green bell pepper, seeded and halved
1 medium yellow onion, peeled and halved
2 whole cloves garlic
1 whole Red Fresno, jalapeño, or serrano pepper
¼ cup watercress leaves
Juice of ½ lime
½ teaspoon ground cumin
1 teaspoon dried oregano
½ teaspoon black pepper
½ teaspoon salt

Preheat the oven to 375°F.

Arrange the tomatoes, bell pepper, onion, garlic, and chili in a round baking pan. Roast for 15 to 20 minutes, until the vegetables are tender. Remove from the heat and let cool slightly.

In a large mixing bowl, place the tomatoes and mash with the back of a spoon. Dice the bell pepper and onion and add them to the tomatoes. Mince the garlic and chili (after removing the seeds) and add them to the vegetables. Blend in the watercress, lime juice, and seasonings and toss well. Serve warm or chill for later.

Makes 4 servings

MANGO-PINEAPPLE CHUTNEY

A well-made chutney runs the continuum of flavors: sweet, tart, hot, and fruity. Chutney, which is rooted in Indian cuisine (where it means "relish") has spread to Britain, the Caribbean, and throughout our country, where it is made with all sorts of fruits. Since the main ingredients are fruit and vinegar, chutney is a naturally low-calorie, low-fat, high-flavor, and zero-cholesterol accompaniment.

1 large mango, peeled, pitted, and chopped
2 cups diced fresh pineapple
1 medium yellow onion, diced
1 large apple (any variety except Red Delicious), diced
1 cup red wine vinegar
½ cup dry white wine or apple juice
½ cup brown sugar, packed
½ cup dark raisins
1 tablespoon minced gingerroot
3 to 4 cloves garlic, minced
1 jalapeño pepper, seeded and minced (optional)
½ teaspoon ground cumin
½ teaspoon ground cloves
¼ teaspoon salt

In a large, nonreactive saucepan, combine all of the ingredients and cook over low heat, stirring occasionally. Simmer for 20 to 30 minutes, until the mixture has a jamlike consistency. Remove from the heat and let stand for 10 minutes.

Serve now or refrigerate for later. If chilled, the chutney will keep for several weeks. Chutney makes a healthful substitute for mayonnaise or butter in a variety of meals: Spoon it over baked potatoes and steamed vegetables, or toss into pasta salads or vegetable curries.

Makes 4 cups

KITCHEN TIPS
- For a change of pace, try a pear, peach, or nectarine in place of the apple.
- When shopping for pineapple, choose one with a faint sweet aroma and one that gives a little when gently pressed.

ARUGULA-SPINACH PESTO

In the twilight of summer, when basil becomes sparse and sorry looking, I like to make a pesto with arugula and spinach. Arugula (known as rocket in Italian) is a tender, leafy herb with a peppery, zippy taste. In the spirit of Garden Pesto Redux (see Index), I've reduced the oil and added a tomato.

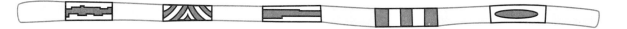

4 cloves garlic
¼ cup pine nuts or unsalted cashews
1 medium tomato, diced
1 cup packed arugula
1 cup packed spinach leaves
¼ cup olive oil
½ teaspoon salt
¼ cup grated Parmesan cheese

In a food processor fitted with a steel blade, add the garlic and nuts and process for 10 to 15 seconds, stopping once to scrape the sides. Add the tomato, arugula, spinach, oil, and salt and process for 15 seconds more, until smooth. Stop at least once to scrape the sides. Transfer to a mixing bowl and fold in the cheese.

Toss the pesto with ½ pound cooked pasta. Or spread over dinner rolls before baking or add 1 to 2 tablespoons with the cheese in Jay's Veggie Burrito (see Index).

Makes about 1 cup

HERB-DIJON VINAIGRETTE

A properly made vinaigrette should strike a fluid balance between the smoothness of oil and the tartness of vinegar. It is a marriage of oil and vinegar, enhanced by mustard and aromatic herbs. A homemade vinaigrette is versatile, easy to prepare, and vastly more rewarding than the sugar-laden, salt-sated, additive-laced commercial dressings on the market.

¼ cup plus 2 tablespoons canola oil
3 tablespoons red wine vinegar
1 tablespoon balsamic vinegar or rice vinegar
1½ teaspoons Dijon mustard
2 teaspoons honey
2 teaspoons mixture of dried herbs including oregano, basil, parsley, and thyme
¼ teaspoon black pepper
¼ teaspoon salt
1 tablespoon chopped basil, parsley, or mint (optional)

In a small mixing bowl, combine all of the ingredients and whisk thoroughly. Refrigerate for 30 minutes to allow the flavors to meld together.

Serve as a dressing for almost any green salad or toss with pasta or rice for a hearty salad.

Makes about ⅔ cup (4 to 6 servings)

KITCHEN TIPS
- For a wilted greens salad, warm the dressing and serve over spinach, dandelion greens, or frisee.

RHUBARB PLUM VINAIGRETTE

Rhubarb is a sadly underrated vegetable (or is it a fruit?). This dressing deliciously illustrates its culinary potential. It is as appealing to the eye as it is to the palate.

> *1 cup unpeeled, diced rhubarb*
> *1 cup unpeeled, diced red or black plums*
> *⅓ cup red wine vinegar*
> *⅓ cup apple juice*
> *1 tablespoon honey*
> *¼ teaspoon black pepper*
> *¼ teaspoon salt*
> *⅓ cup canola oil*

In a small, nonreactive saucepan, place all of the ingredients and cook for 10 to 15 minutes over medium heat, stirring occasionally. Set aside and let cool slightly.

Transfer the mixture to a food processor fitted with a steel blade or to a blender. Blend for about 10 seconds, until smooth. Refrigerate for at least 1 hour before serving.

Place the dressing over a salad of mixed leafy greens.

Makes about 2 cups

GOLDEN PEACH NUTMEG VINAIGRETTE

Here is a luscious way to offer a reduced-fat salad dressing while enjoying the natural sweetness of summer fruit. Nectarines may be used instead of peaches, if desired.

> *4 medium-size ripe peaches, peeled and*
>   *diced*
> *⅓ cup red wine vinegar*
> *⅓ cup apple juice*
> *⅓ cup canola oil*
> *1 tablespoon honey*
> *½ teaspoon black pepper*
> *¼ teaspoon nutmeg*
> *¼ teaspoon salt*

In a blender or a food processor fitted with a steel blade, place all of the ingredients and process for 10 to 15 seconds, until the dressing is creamy. Transfer to a serving pitcher and serve with a mixed green salad or refrigerate for later.

Makes 2 cups (12 to 16 servings)

TROPICAL MANGO BARBECUE SAUCE

This fruity table sauce makes a savory accompaniment to rice and beans, baked potatoes, roasted plantains, baked tofu, or vegetables on the grill.

1 ripe mango, peeled, pitted, and chopped
1 medium yellow onion, diced
1 medium carrot, peeled and diced
½ Scotch bonnet or 1 jalapeño pepper,
  seeded and chopped
2 cloves garlic, chopped
1 cup red wine vinegar
½ cup pineapple juice
2 tablespoons Worcestershire sauce
⅓ cup brown sugar, packed
½ teaspoon salt
½ teaspoon allspice

In a large, nonreactive saucepan, combine all of the ingredients and cook over low heat, stirring occasionally. Simmer for 20 to 25 minutes, until the mixture has a jamlike consistency.

Allow the sauce to cool to room temperature. In a food processor fitted with a steel blade, place the mixture and process for 15 to 20 seconds. The sauce should be smooth, with a few chunks. If refrigerated, the sauce should keep for several weeks.

Makes about 2½ cups

CRANBERRY FRUIT CHUTNEY

The cranberry is one of those rare fruits that is at home in both sweet and savory surroundings. This tangy chutney is a popular condiment on my Thanksgiving menu. It is far more appealing than those canned, mass-produced, processed-tasting jiggling cylinders of jelly masquerading as cranberry relish.

> 12 ounces fresh or frozen cranberries
> 1 large unpeeled apple (any variety except Red Delicious), diced
> 1 large unpeeled Bosc pear, diced
> 1 large yellow onion, diced
> 4 cloves garlic, minced
> 1 tablespoon minced gingerroot
> ¾ cup brown sugar, packed
> ½ cup dark raisins or 1 cup chopped dried apricots
> 1½ cups red wine vinegar
> 1 cup apple juice or apple cider
> ½ teaspoon black pepper
> ½ teaspoon ground cumin
> ½ teaspoon salt
> ¼ teaspoon ground cloves

In a large, nonreactive saucepan, combine all of the ingredients and cook over low heat, stirring occasionally, for 25 to 30 minutes, until the mixture has a jamlike consistency. Allow the chutney to cool to room temperature. Serve now or refrigerate for later. If refrigerated, the chutney should keep for several weeks.

Makes 6 to 8 servings

TAHINI YOGURT DRESSING

A friend of mine, attempting to eat more healthfully, began eating tossed salads for lunch. So far, so good. Unfortunately, he buried his salads in super high-calorie creamy blue cheese dressing. As an alternative, I suggested this lighter "creamy" dressing, and since then, his addiction to blue cheese has ended.

> 1 cup plain low-fat yogurt
> ¼ cup tahini (sesame seed paste)
> Juice of 1 lemon
> 1 large clove garlic, minced
> 2 tablespoons minced fresh parsley (or 1 tablespoon dried)
> ¼ teaspoon black pepper
> ¼ teaspoon salt

In a small mixing bowl, whisk all of the ingredients. Refrigerate for 1 hour to allow the flavors to meld together. Serve as a salad dressing, vegetable dip, or sandwich spread.

Makes 6 to 8 servings

MINT LEAF–COCONUT CHUTNEY

This is a natural cooling condiment for spicy Indian curries, especially Sweet Potato and Broccoli Sambar (see Index). My friend, Dr. Helena Das, who recently toured India, contributed to this recipe.

> 1 cup shredded coconut (unsweetened, if
>   possible)
> 2 to 3 tablespoons chopped mint leaves
> 2 teaspoons minced gingerroot
> ¾ teaspoon paprika
> ⅛ teaspoon cayenne pepper
> ½ cup plain low-fat yogurt
> 1 teaspoon fresh lemon juice

In a small mixing bowl, combine all of the ingredients and blend well. Transfer to a serving bowl and chill for 1 hour before serving, allowing the flavors to mingle.

Makes 4 to 6 servings

BLACK BEAN SOFRITO

Sofrito is a multipurpose sauce found on Puerto Rican and Spanish tables. It is a tasty way to jazz up a plain rice dish at the last minute. When I'm in the mood for cross-cultural fusion cooking, I serve it over Pimiento Polenta (see Index).

> 1 tablespoon canola oil
> 1 medium yellow onion, diced
> 1 medium green bell pepper, seeded and
>   diced
> 2 cloves garlic, minced
> 1 15-ounce can black beans, drained
> 1 15-ounce can stewed tomatoes
> ½ teaspoon ground cumin
> ½ teaspoon black pepper
> ½ teaspoon salt
> 2 tablespoons chopped cilantro

In a medium saucepan, heat the oil. Add the onion, bell pepper, and garlic and sauté for 5 to 7 minutes. Add the beans, tomatoes, and dry seasonings and cook for 7 to 10 minutes more over low heat, stirring frequently. Stir in the cilantro and remove from the heat. Spoon over rice or other grain dishes.

Makes 6 servings

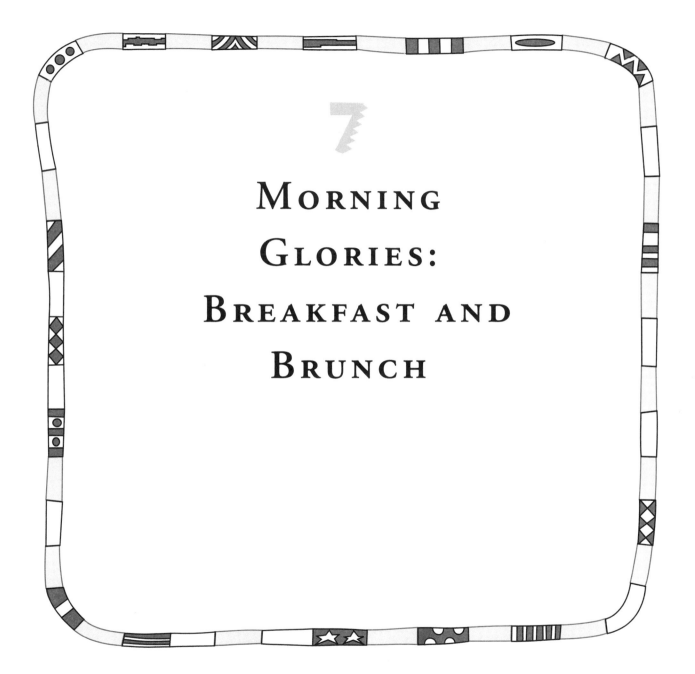

7

MORNING
GLORIES:
BREAKFAST AND
BRUNCH

reakfast is widely thought to be the most important meal of the day. Naturally, it should not be squandered on energy-zapping, excessively fatty foods (or worse, skipped altogether). Although I gave up lumberjack breakfasts with bacon and sausage years ago, the memory of those monster caloric meals—and subsequent bouts with lethargy and sluggishness—still lingers. Breakfast is an occasion to charge up the body with energy for the day ahead, not drain it.

On most days my breakfast is a bowl of bran flakes mixed with oatmeal and wheat and barley cereal, topped with banana. It's a form of high-fiber gruel. But on the weekends and on special occasions, breakfast and brunch are times to have fun and indulge. This chapter offers the unexpected: Zucchini Crepes, filled with pureed apples; Spinach Spuds, which liven up the standard fare of home fries; Pumpkin Buckwheat Pancakes Filled with Fruit; Banana Bread French Toast; and grilled Monte Cristo with Seitan (a high-protein meat substitute). There is also a taste of the exotic with Costa Rican Gallo Pinto and Egyptian Ful Medames.

There are a few tricks to preparing a heart-smart breakfast. For starters, egg whites and egg substitutes can replace all or most of the eggs normally used. Adding seasonal fruit to pancakes and waffles and using buttermilk in recipes calling for milk or cream further lightens the load. Last night's vegetables and fresh herbs can rejuvenate home fries, roasted potatoes, and crepes. In this chapter, you'll see that it is possible to create healthful morning food, retain the spirit of breakfast, and eliminate the meat, greasy fries, and empty-calorie griddle fare oozing with butter.

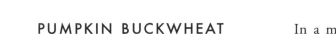

PUMPKIN BUCKWHEAT PANCAKES FILLED WITH FRUIT

It is always a special morning in my house when pancakes are on the menu. There is something intrinsically gratifying about the smell of pancakes cooking on a hot griddle and fresh coffee brewing in the kitchen. These pumpkin and fruit griddle cakes are light, healthful, and easy to prepare.

1½ cups buckwheat flour
½ cup unbleached wheat flour
¼ cup brown sugar, packed
2 teaspoons baking powder
1 teaspoon salt
½ teaspoon allspice
1 large egg and 1 large egg white, beaten
2 cups buttermilk or skim milk
1 cup mashed pumpkin
4 apples (any variety except Red Delicious),
  peaches, or nectarines, seeded and chopped
Vegetable spray

In a medium mixing bowl, combine the dry ingredients. In another medium bowl, whisk the egg, buttermilk, and pumpkin together. Fold the liquid ingredients into the dry ingredients and beat until the batter is fluid and free of lumps.

Preheat a lightly sprayed griddle or skillet. Ladle about ½ cup of the batter onto the griddle, forming a pancake about 7 inches wide. Sprinkle about 2 tablespoons of the chopped fruit evenly over the pancake. Flip after 3 to 4 minutes (when the edges begin to brown). Continue cooking until the pancake is golden brown. Remove to a warm plate and repeat the process with the remaining batter.

Serve the pancakes with real maple syrup and freshly brewed coffee.

Makes 8 pancakes

BANANA BREAD FRENCH TOAST

I discovered this fabulous brunch idea at the Villa Banfi dining room of the Statler Hotel at Cornell University, my alma mater. Here is my version.

½ cup egg substitutes (about 2 eggs, beaten)
8 slices Hazelnut Banana Bread (see Index)
* or your favorite banana bread*
Vegetable spray

In a shallow mixing bowl, pour the egg substitutes or eggs.

Heat a lightly sprayed nonstick skillet over medium heat. Take a slice of banana bread and dredge both sides in the egg mixture. Place onto the heated skillet and cook both sides until golden brown. Transfer to warm plates and repeat with the remaining slices of bread.

If you'd like, serve with Nutmeg Applesauce (see Index).

Makes 4 servings

ROSEMARY ROASTED SWEET POTATOES

I have a penchant for sweet potatoes—never, never the canned stuff, but the portly roots straight from the earth. Roasting brings out their natural sweetness.

4 cloves garlic, minced
2 tablespoons olive oil or canola oil
3 to 4 tablespoons chopped rosemary leaves
½ teaspoon salt
¼ teaspoon cayenne pepper
4 medium unpeeled sweet potatoes, scrubbed
* and diced*
1 teaspoon paprika

Preheat the oven to 375°F.

In a small mixing bowl, combine the garlic, oil, rosemary, salt, cayenne, and potatoes and toss together. Let stand for 5 minutes.

Place the potatoes on a greased baking pan. Lightly sprinkle the paprika over the potatoes. Bake for 35 to 40 minutes or until the potatoes are easily pierced by a fork. Serve immediately.

Makes 4 servings

SPINACH SPUDS

I have fond memories of my father taking me to a local diner on Saturdays for breakfast when I was young. I had a ravenous appetite and frequently cleaned off the home fries from his plate as well as mine. To this day I still love potatoes in the morning, but without the bacon drippings and fat. The fresh spinach used here is a healthful alternative.

4 cups unpeeled, diced white potatoes
1 tablespoon canola oil
1 small medium onion, chopped fine
2 cloves garlic, minced
2 cups chopped spinach, packed
2 scallions, chopped
1 teaspoon paprika
½ teaspoon salt
¼ teaspoon cayenne pepper
1 to 2 teaspoons bottled hot sauce (optional)

In a medium saucepan, place the potatoes in enough boiling water to cover and cook for about 15 minutes, until tender. Drain in a colander and cool slightly.

In a medium skillet, heat the oil. Add the onion and garlic and sauté for about 5 minutes. Stir in the potatoes, spinach, scallions, seasonings, and bottled hot sauce, if desired, and cook for 5 to 7 minutes over low heat, stirring frequently. Serve hot with ketchup on the side.

Makes 4 servings

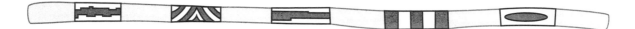

HERB CREPES WITH SUMMER BERRIES

This is a morning celebration of summer's finest fruits and herbs.

FOR THE CREPES:

1¼ cups buttermilk
*1 large egg and 1 large egg white, beaten
    (or ½ cup egg substitutes)*
3 to 4 tablespoons canola oil
½ teaspoon salt
1 cup unbleached all-purpose flour
*¼ cup chopped mixed basil, mint, or
    tarragon*
Vegetable spray

FOR THE FILLING:

2 medium bananas, peeled and sliced
1 cup slivered strawberries or raspberries
1 cup blueberries
1 cup vanilla low-fat yogurt
1 cup low-fat granola
¼ teaspoon ground nutmeg

First, make the crepe batter: in a large mixing bowl, whisk together the buttermilk, eggs, oil, and salt. Blend in the flour and herbs and refrigerate the batter for 15 to 30 minutes.

Lightly spray a 9-inch crepe pan or nonstick skillet and ladle about ½ cup of batter into the pan. Tilt the pan to ease the batter around the base of the pan, forming a thin, round pancake. When the edges of the crepe are light brown, flip the crepe with a smooth motion. Continue cooking until the surface is light brown and then remove to a warm plate. Cook the remaining batter in the same fashion and stack the finished crepes on top of each other.

For the filling, toss the bananas, berries, yogurt, granola, and nutmeg in a mixing bowl. Fill each crepe with about ½ cup of the fruit mixture, forming a log in the middle and wrapping the crepe around the filling (like a burrito). Serve immediately.

Makes 6 servings

ZUCCHINI CREPES WITH APPLE FILLING

The crepe has the potential to be a stuffy dish, but adding shredded zucchini makes it fun. Here are some crepe-making tips: Always start with a sizzling hot pan, and when it is time for the turn, flip the crepe with one smooth motion. Do not be discouraged by the first crepe—its purpose is to season the pan. Return to the charge and try again.

FOR THE CREPES:

1¼ cups buttermilk
1 large egg and 1 large egg white, beaten
  (or ½ cup egg substitutes)
3 to 4 tablespoons canola oil
½ teaspoon salt
1 cup unbleached all-purpose flour
1 cup shredded zucchini
Vegetable spray

FOR THE FILLING:

¼ cup water
10 to 12 apples (any variety except Red
  Delicious), peeled and chopped
2 tablespoons honey
½ teaspoon cinnamon
1 cup plain low-fat yogurt (optional)

First, make the crepe batter: in a large mixing bowl, whisk together the buttermilk, eggs, oil, and salt. Blend in the flour and zucchini and refrigerate the batter for 15 to 30 minutes.

Meanwhile, make the apple filling: in a medium saucepan, place the water and apples and cook over medium heat for 20 to 25 minutes, stirring occasionally, until the apples have a mashed consistency. Stir in the honey and spice and mash the apples against the side of the pan with a wooden spoon.

To cook the crepes, heat a lightly sprayed 9-inch crepe pan or skillet and ladle about ½ cup of batter into the pan. Tilt the pan to ease the batter around the base of the pan, forming a thin, round pancake. When the edges of the crepe are golden brown, flip the crepe with a smooth motion. Continue cooking until the remaining surface is golden brown and then remove to a warm plate. Cook the remaining batter in the same fashion and stack the finished crepes on top of each other.

To fill the crepes, place each crepe on a serving plate and spoon about 1 cup of the mashed apples in the center. Wrap the crepe around the filling and roll tight. If desired, spoon a dollop of yogurt over the top of each crepe.

Makes 6 servings

OMELET MEDITERRANEO

One Sunday, while jogging uphill in a five-mile race and trying to keep my spirits up, I dreamed about making this omelet immediately after the run. I finished the race in a modest time but the omelet turned out to be the real winner.

1 small red or green bell pepper, seeded and
  chopped
1 medium tomato, diced
2 cloves garlic, minced
¼ cup pitted black olives, sliced
2 scallions, chopped
1 cup egg substitutes or 4 large eggs, beaten
2 tablespoons skim milk
1 tablespoon mixture of dried oregano, basil,
  marjoram, and thyme
Vegetable spray
2 to 3 ounces crumbled feta cheese

In a small mixing bowl, combine the pepper, tomato, garlic, olives, and scallions. Set aside.

In another small bowl, whisk together the eggs, milk, and herbs. Heat a lightly sprayed nonstick skillet or omelet pan and pour about one-half of the egg mixture into the skillet. Swirl to the edges of the pan. Reduce the heat and cook for 1 to 2 minutes; then slide a spatula underneath the omelet to ease the excess mixture onto the pan's surface.

When the omelet is light brown around the edges and the top surface is barely moist, add one-half of the vegetable mixture to one-half of the omelet, forming a half moon. Add about 1 tablespoon of the cheese to the mixture and gently fold over the other half of the omelet. Cover the pan and cook for about 1 minute more; then turn off the heat. Let the omelet sit in the pan for another minute and then slide onto a warm plate.

Re-season the pan with vegetable spray and repeat the process with the remaining ingredients. Serve with Rosemary Roasted Sweet Potatoes or Spinach Spuds (see Index for recipes).

Makes 2 servings

BREAKFAST BURRITO

The idea of wrapping skillet eggs in a flour tortilla provides a nice change of pace.

Vegetable spray
1 medium red bell pepper, seeded and diced
4 to 6 medium button mushrooms, sliced
2 scallions, chopped
½ cup corn kernels, fresh or frozen and
  thawed
2 tablespoons chopped cilantro
½ teaspoon ground cumin

½ teaspoon black pepper
¼ teaspoon salt
½ cup egg substitutes (about 2 eggs, beaten)
¼ cup shredded low-fat provolone or Swiss
   cheese
2 10-inch flour tortillas

Heat a lightly sprayed nonstick skillet. Add the pepper, mushrooms, and scallions and sauté for 5 to 7 minutes. Stir in the corn and seasonings and cook for 2 to 3 minutes more. Whisk in the eggs and cook over medium heat, stirring frequently. When the eggs are completely cooked (fluffy, not brown), remove from the heat and fold in the cheese.

Warm the tortillas over a burner or pan and then place on 2 plates. Spoon the egg mixture into the center of each tortilla, forming logs. Roll the tortilla around the mixture and serve with Salsa! Salsa! or a favorite salsa. Rosemary Roasted Sweet Potatoes, Black Bean Sofrito, or Spinach Spuds (see Index for recipes) make good side dishes.

Makes 2 servings

GALLO PINTO

If you ever visit Costa Rica, you will discover *gallo pinto*, their national dish. It is a rice and bean meal, spiced up here for a real "power" breakfast. Gallo pinto (it means "painted rooster") is often served with Costa Rican Cabbage Salad (see Index) and a Worcestershire-like table condiment called Salsa Linzano.

1 tablespoon canola oil
1 small yellow onion, chopped
1 medium red bell pepper, seeded and diced
1 to 2 cloves garlic, minced
4 cups cooked long-grain brown or white
   rice
1 15-ounce can black beans, drained
1 teaspoon dried oregano
½ teaspoon ground cumin
Worcestershire sauce, to taste
Salt and black pepper, to taste

In a large nonstick skillet, heat the oil. Add the onion, pepper, and garlic and sauté for about 5 minutes, until the vegetables are tender. Add the cooked rice, beans, and seasonings except salt and pepper and cook over medium heat for about 10 minutes, stirring frequently, until the rice and beans are completely reheated. Stir in a few drops of the Worcestershire sauce. Serve at once.

Pass the bottle of Worcestershire sauce at the table and add salt and pepper to taste.

Makes 4 servings

EGYPTIAN FUL MEDAMES

Ful medames is served everywhere in Egypt, from street-side vendors to elegant restaurants. Traditionally, the beans are "buried" beneath the eggs and spices. The fava beans in Egypt are smaller than those grown in Europe. They are available in the specialty sections of well-stocked supermarkets.

> 1 18-ounce can small fava beans, drained
> 1 teaspoon ground cumin
> 2 cloves garlic, minced
> 4 small hard-boiled eggs, peeled
> 1 tablespoon minced parsley
> 1 lemon, quartered
> 2 to 3 tablespoons olive oil
> Salt and black pepper, to taste

In a small saucepan, heat the beans until steaming. Transfer the beans to a bowl and stir in the cumin and garlic.

Place the hard-boiled eggs in the center of 4 individual soup bowls. Spoon the beans over the eggs to cover. Sprinkle the parsley over the beans and then squeeze a wedge of lemon over each bowl. Mash the beans and egg together and then drizzle less than 1 tablespoon of oil over each dish. Season with salt and pepper.

Makes 4 servings

ARTICHOKE AND WHITE BEAN FRITTATA

Frittata is a rustic Italian potato-egg dish. This version has a down-home look with a sophisticated flavor.

> 2 cups peeled, diced white potatoes
> 1 tablespoon canola oil
> 1 small yellow onion, diced
> 1 medium red bell pepper, seeded and diced
> 4 scallions, chopped
> 1 8-ounce can artichoke hearts, rinsed, drained, and chopped coarse
> 1 15-ounce can white kidney beans, drained
> 2 tablespoons chopped fresh parsley (or 1 tablespoon dried)
> 1 teaspoon dried oregano
> 1 cup egg substitutes (or 4 large eggs, beaten)
> ½ cup shredded low-fat Swiss cheese or part-skim mozzarella
> Salt and black pepper, to taste

In a small saucepan, place the potatoes in enough boiling water to cover and cook for about 15 minutes, until tender. Drain in a colander and cool slightly.

In a large nonstick skillet or Dutch oven, heat the oil. Add the onion and bell pepper and sauté for about 5 minutes. Add the potatoes,

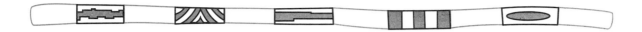

scallions, artichoke hearts, and beans and cook for about 5 minutes more, stirring occasionally.

Meanwhile, whisk the herbs together with the eggs. Reduce the heat to low and pour the egg mixture into the pan, blending the eggs into the vegetables. Sprinkle the cheese over the top, cover, and cook on low for 4 to 5 minutes. Let stand for 5 minutes more before serving.

Season with salt and pepper to taste and serve with whole-wheat toast or English muffins.

Makes 4 servings

MONTE CRISTO WITH SEITAN

This egg-dipped sandwich is normally made with sliced ham, but seitan, a gluten product made from wheat, makes an excellent substitute for the meat.

½ cup egg substitutes
¼ pound low-fat Swiss cheese, sliced thin
8 slices whole-wheat bread
½ pound seitan, sliced
Vegetable spray

In a shallow bowl, add the egg substitutes.

Make 4 sandwiches: lay the cheese slices on 4 slices of bread, then cover with a layer of seitan, then a slice of cheese. Cover each with a slice of bread.

Heat a lightly sprayed nonstick skillet. Dredge both sides of one of the sandwiches in the egg batter and place on the heated skillet. Cook both sides until golden brown. Repeat with remaining sandwiches.

Makes 4 servings

KITCHEN TIPS
- Seitan is available in the refrigerator section of well-stocked natural food stores.

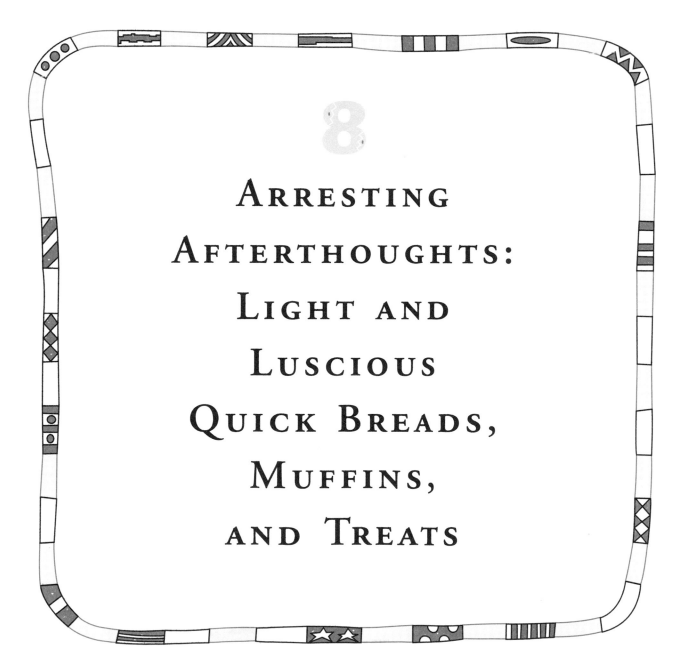

8

ARRESTING
AFTERTHOUGHTS:
LIGHT AND
LUSCIOUS
QUICK BREADS,
MUFFINS,
AND TREATS

t's a common scenario: we eat a properly healthful and well-balanced meal—then, after a brief moment of righteous contemplation, plow into a decadent dessert. This is payback for good behavior. We surrender to temptation and submerge our taste buds in a river of chocolate, savoring every mouthful. Then the hangover of guilt sets in, unwanted calories pile up, and the postmortem begins: where did our willpower go? Next time, things *will* be different . . .

Americans have a love-hate relationship with sweets. But here's the good news: there are clever ways to have your cake and eat it, too, to indulge without sacrificing taste. The recipes in this chapter replace most of the fat in muffins and cookies with applesauce, apple juice, or orange juice. Low-fat milk and buttermilk replace milk or cream. Creative uses for tofu, soy milk, and rice milk also offer hope for happier endings.

Dessert is an opportunity to include naturally sweet fruits in the meal. Here you'll find recipes for apples, cranberries, bananas, peaches, berries, mangoes, and other fruits. In addition, vitamin-rich pumpkin, sweet potatoes, winter squash, carrots, zucchini, and corn inspire resourceful treats. Wholesome grains such as bran, oatmeal, rice, and cornmeal make welcome appearances as well.

The road to healthful eating is indeed lined with confectionery pitfalls and chocolate roadblocks. The mere sight of dessert elicits passion and pang, desire and conflict. Yet, with a few alterations, your health-minded compass will remain pointed in the right direction as you savor every indulgent morsel of your well-deserved dessert.

ZUCCHINI CORN BREAD

Creating a low-fat corn bread that was still moist and desirable was a daunting task, but not an insurmountable one. This wholesome treat is fortified with moist shredded zucchini.

1 cup yellow cornmeal
1 cup unbleached all-purpose flour
⅓ cup sugar
1 tablespoon baking powder
½ teaspoon salt
1 large egg plus 1 large egg white, beaten
1 cup buttermilk
2 tablespoons canola oil
*1 cup corn kernels, fresh or frozen and
    thawed*
1 cup shredded zucchini
Vegetable spray

Preheat the oven to 375°F.

In a medium mixing bowl, combine the cornmeal, flour, sugar, baking powder, and salt. In a small bowl, whisk together the eggs, buttermilk, and oil. Gently fold the liquid ingredients into the dry ingredients until a batter is formed. Fold in the corn and zucchini.

Pour the batter into a lightly sprayed 8-inch square or round baking pan. Bake for 20 to 25 minutes, until the crust is lightly browned and a toothpick inserted in the center comes out clean. Remove from the heat and let cool for a few minutes before cutting. Serve warm.

Makes 10 to 12 servings

CHILI CORN BREAD

Chili peppers and pimientos add spice to this corn bread, and corn kernels supply additional moisture.

> 1 cup yellow cornmeal
> 1 cup unbleached all-purpose flour
> ¼ cup sugar
> 1 tablespoon baking powder
> ½ teaspoon salt
> 1 large egg plus 1 large egg white, beaten
> 1 cup buttermilk
> ¼ cup canola oil
> 2 tablespoons chopped pimientos
> 2 to 3 jalapeño peppers, seeded and minced
> 1 cup corn kernels, fresh or frozen and
>   thawed
> 4 scallions, chopped
> Vegetable spray

Preheat the oven to 375°F.

Combine the cornmeal, flour, sugar, baking powder, and salt in a mixing bowl. In a separate bowl, whisk together the eggs, buttermilk, oil, pimientos, peppers, corn, and scallions. Gently fold the liquid ingredients into the dry ingredients until the mixture forms a batter.

Pour the batter into a sprayed 9-inch round baking pan. Bake for 20 to 25 minutes, until the crust is lightly browned and a toothpick inserted in the center comes out clean. Remove from the heat and let cool for a few minutes. Cut into wedges and serve warm.

Makes 8 to 10 servings

ZUCCHINI-CARROT HEALTH MUFFINS

I first prepared these muffins for a Healthy Heart cooking class I was teaching and they won mega-kudos from the students. Orange juice replaces most of the oil that would typically be used, and the carrots and zucchini add valuable vitamins and minerals.

> ½ cup canola oil
> ½ cup orange juice
> 1 cup brown sugar, packed
> 1 large egg plus 1 large egg white, beaten
> 1 teaspoon vanilla extract
> 2 cups unbleached all-purpose flour
> 1 tablespoon baking powder
> 1 teaspoon salt
> 1 teaspoon cinnamon
> 1 teaspoon ground nutmeg
> 1 cup grated zucchini
> 1 cup peeled, grated carrot
> ½ cup dark raisins or 1 cup diced walnuts
> Vegetable spray

Preheat the oven to 350°F.

In a small mixing bowl, whisk together the oil, juice, and sugar. Add the eggs and vanilla extract and continue whisking until the batter is light. In a medium bowl, combine the dry ingredients. Gently fold the dry ingredients into the liquid ingredients, forming a batter. Gently fold in zucchini, carrot, and raisins or walnuts.

Pour the batter into a sprayed muffin tin and bake for 20 to 25 minutes, until a toothpick inserted in the center comes out clean. Remove from the heat and let cool for a few minutes. Serve warm.

Makes 10 to 12 muffins

HAZELNUT BANANA BREAD

This banana bread is lighter and nuttier than most banana breads. Use overripe bananas for the best results. If your bananas are overripe before you are ready to make the bread, you can save them in the freezer.

½ cup canola oil
½ cup orange juice
1 cup brown sugar, packed
1 large egg plus 1 large egg white
¼ cup buttermilk or skim milk
1 teaspoon vanilla extract

2 cups mashed ripe bananas (4 to 5 bananas)
2 cups unbleached all-purpose flour
1 teaspoon nutmeg
1 teaspoon cinnamon
1 teaspoon baking powder
½ teaspoon salt
1 cup chopped hazelnuts or walnuts
Vegetable spray

Preheat the oven to 350°F.

In a medium mixing bowl, whisk together the oil, juice, and sugar. Add the eggs, buttermilk, and vanilla and whisk until the batter is light. Blend in the bananas.

In a small bowl, mix the dry ingredients. Gently fold the dry ingredients into the banana batter. Spoon the batter into two 8½″ × 4½″ sprayed loaf pans and bake for 40 to 50 minutes, until a toothpick inserted in the center comes out clean. Let cool for about 15 minutes on a rack before serving.

Makes 2 small loaves

KITCHEN TIPS
- Day-old banana bread makes excellent French toast (see Index for recipe).

PUMPKIN BRAN MEGA-MUFFINS

For years the bran muffins I sampled were dry, tasteless, and universally disappointing. They may have been healthful, but I never finished them. With this in mind, I aspired to create a moist, nutritious, good-tasting bran muffin. This version, enriched with pumpkin, molasses, and applesauce, is the enlightened result.

½ cup canola oil
½ cup applesauce
½ cup low-fat milk or buttermilk
¾ cup brown sugar, packed
1 large egg plus 1 large egg white
¼ cup dark molasses
2 cups mashed pumpkin
1 cup dark raisins
2 cups wheat bran (unprocessed)
½ cup unbleached all-purpose flour
1½ teaspoons baking powder
1 teaspoon cinnamon
½ teaspoon salt
Vegetable spray

Preheat the oven to 375°F.

In a medium mixing bowl, whisk together the oil, applesauce, milk, and sugar. Add the eggs and molasses and whisk until the batter is light. Blend in the mashed pumpkin and raisins.

In a medium bowl, mix the dry ingredients. Gently fold the dry ingredients into the pumpkin batter. Spoon the batter into lightly sprayed muffin tins and bake for 40 to 50 minutes, until a toothpick inserted in the center comes out clean.

Let cool for about 10 minutes on a rack before serving.

Makes 6 mega-muffins or about 12 small muffins

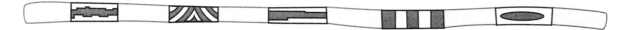

SWEET POTATO–MOLASSES MUFFINS

These sweet potato muffins, partially sweetened with molasses, are an excellent way to sneak a beta-carotene rich snack into your meal plan. You may not be able to eat just one! The raw, untamed flavor of molasses comes through here with satisfying subtlety.

2 large sweet potatoes, halved
½ cup canola oil
½ cup brown sugar, packed
½ cup dark molasses
2 large eggs or ½ cup egg substitutes
½ cup skim milk or buttermilk
1 teaspoon vanilla extract
2 cups unbleached all-purpose flour
1 tablespoon baking powder
1 teaspoon salt
1 teaspoon cinnamon
½ teaspoon nutmeg or allspice
½ cup dark raisins or 1 cup diced pecans or
walnuts

In a medium saucepan, place the potatoes in enough boiling water to cover and cook over medium heat for about 20 minutes, until tender. Drain in a colander and cool under cold running water. Remove skin. Transfer the potatoes to a bowl and mash with the back of a large spoon or potato masher.

Preheat the oven to 375°F.

In a medium mixing bowl, beat the oil, sugar, and molasses together until light. Blend in the eggs, milk, and vanilla. Blend in the sweet potatoes.

In a small bowl, mix the flour, baking powder, salt, and spices. Gently fold the dry ingredients into the sweet potato batter. Fold in the raisins (or walnuts). Spoon the batter into greased muffin tins and bake for 25 to 30 minutes or until a toothpick inserted in the center comes out clean. Remove from the pan and let cool on a rack for 10 minutes before serving.

Makes 12 to 14 muffins or 6 mega-muffins

MANGO AND BANANA FLAMBÉ

Flambé is usually prepared with a buttery sauce, but apple juice makes a great low-fat replacement. Other fruits such as kiwi, strawberries, and peaches may also be used.

¼ cup apple juice
2 tablespoons brown sugar, packed
1 large ripe mango, peeled, pitted, and
*   sliced*
3 to 4 bananas, peeled and sliced crosswise
¼ teaspoon cinnamon or allspice
¼ cup dark rum
Splash of banana liqueur (optional)
1 pint low-fat frozen yogurt

In a medium skillet, combine the apple juice and brown sugar and cook over medium heat for about 3 minutes, stirring frequently. Add the mango, bananas, and cinnamon and cook for 3 to 4 minutes more. Turn the slices gently, coating them with the juice mixture.

Remove the pan from the heat and add the rum and liqueur, if desired. Return to the heat and bring to a simmer over medium heat. Carefully touch a lighted match to the pan, flambéing the fruit. Allow the flame to subside and continue cooking for 1 minute more.

Spoon the fruit over low-fat frozen yogurt.

Makes 4 servings

KITCHEN TIPS
- When flambéing, never pour liquor directly from the bottle into the pan. Always measure out the liquor and transfer it to a small pitcher.

NUTMEG APPLESAUCE

Every October in Ithaca my friends and I make our yearly pilgrimage to the area's orchards for an afternoon of apple picking. For days afterward a blizzard of apple dishes ensues. This is one of the simplest and most satisfying apple creations. If you make a large batch, place the apples in a bowl of cold water with a few slices of lemon as you dice them. The acidified water keeps them from browning.

8 unpeeled apples (any variety except Red
*   Delicious), diced*
4 to 5 tablespoons water
2 tablespoons honey
½ teaspoon nutmeg or allspice

In a medium saucepan, place the apples and water and cook over medium heat for 25 to 30 minutes, stirring occasionally, until the apples have a mashed consistency. Stir in the honey and nutmeg. Let the mixture cool for a few minutes.

Transfer the mashed apples to a blender and mix until smooth. (For a chunky sauce, mash the apples with a spoon by hand.) Chill for at least 1 hour before serving.

Makes 4 cups

CRANBERRY BOG OATMEAL COOKIES

Cranberries are at home in both sweet and savory surroundings. The glistening berries provide a burst of flavor in these chewy oatmeal and walnut cookies. Applesauce replaces half of the fat typically called for.

4 tablespoons margarine, softened
1 cup brown sugar, packed
½ cup applesauce
1 large egg
2 tablespoons molasses
2 tablespoons water
1 teaspoon vanilla extract
2 cups rolled oatmeal
1 cup unbleached all-purpose flour
½ teaspoon cinnamon
½ teaspoon nutmeg
½ teaspoon salt
½ teaspoon baking powder
1 cup cranberries
½ cup diced walnuts

In a large mixing bowl or mixer, blend the margarine and sugar together until light. Beat in the applesauce, egg, molasses, water, and vanilla.

In a medium bowl, mix together the dry ingredients. Gently fold the dry ingredients into the wet ingredients. Fold in the cranberries and walnuts. Cover and chill the dough for 30 minutes.

Preheat the oven to 375°F.

Using an ice cream scooper, scoop the dough onto a lightly greased cookie sheet. Bake for about 20 minutes, until lightly brown. Cool on a rack for 10 minutes before serving.

Makes about 12 cookies

J.J.'S FAMOUS CHOCOLATE CHIP WALNUT COOKIES

Fresh out of college, before I became a chef, I started a cookie business. I baked and delivered over 120 dozen cookies a day, every day. Cookies were my life, and at times it seemed the whole town clamored for these delicious homemade treats.

Here, then, is the recipe that launched my culinary career, without any revisions.

2 sticks margarine, softened (1 cup)
¾ cup brown sugar, packed
¾ cup sugar
2 large eggs
1 teaspoon water
1 teaspoon vanilla extract
2½ cups unbleached all-purpose flour
½ teaspoon salt
1 teaspoon baking powder
1½ to 2 cups diced walnuts
12 ounces semisweet chocolate chips

In a large mixing bowl or mixer, blend the margarine and sugars together until light. Blend in the eggs one at a time, and beat until the batter is creamy. Blend in the water and vanilla.

In a medium bowl, mix together the dry ingredients. Gently fold the dry ingredients into the wet ingredients. Fold in the walnuts and chocolate chips. Cover and chill the dough for 30 minutes to 1 hour.

Preheat the oven to 375°F.

Using an ice cream scooper, scoop the dough onto a greased cookie sheet. Bake for about 20 minutes, until lightly brown. Cool on a rack for 10 minutes before serving.

Makes about 12 large or 20 small cookies

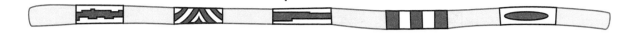

CHAYOTE CARROT BREAD

Chayote is a pale green, pear-shaped squash used in Caribbean and Creole cooking. The firm, white, moist flesh can be shredded and added to sweet quick breads like zucchini. Chayote is also called christophene, mirliton, and cho cho.

½ cup canola oil
½ cup orange juice
⅓ cup sugar
2 large egg whites plus 1 large egg
1 teaspoon vanilla extract
2 cups grated chayote (2 to 3 squash)
1 cup peeled, grated carrot
2 cups unbleached all-purpose flour
2 teaspoons baking soda
1 teaspoon baking powder
1 teaspoon salt
1 teaspoon cinnamon
1 teaspoon nutmeg
1 cup diced walnuts (optional)
Vegetable spray

Preheat the oven to 350°F.

In a large mixing bowl, whisk together the oil, juice, and sugar. Add the eggs and whisk until the batter is light and creamy. Fold in the remaining ingredients and blend well. Pour the batter into 12 lightly sprayed mini-loaf pans and bake for about 25 minutes, until a toothpick inserted in the center comes out clean. Serve warm.

Makes 12 small loaves

KITCHEN TIPS
• Chayote is available in Caribbean and Latin American specialty stores and in produce sections of well-stocked supermarkets.

CHOCOLATE MOCHA TOFU CHEESECAKE

For this decadent cheesecake, tofu replaces half of the cheese typically called for, and egg whites are used instead of whole eggs. If you harbor reservations about tofu, this invention might be a coming of age for your taste buds. The trick to cooking with tofu is to pair it with strongly flavored ingredients such as chocolate.

FOR THE PIE CRUST:

About ⅓ pound graham crackers, crushed
2 tablespoons margarine
1 large egg white

FOR THE CHEESECAKE:

1 cup semisweet chocolate chips
¼ cup coffee liqueur (Kahlua or Tia Maria)
½ pound firm tofu
½ pound part-skim ricotta cheese
¼ cup sugar
2 large egg whites
2 to 3 tablespoons diced walnuts (optional)

Preheat the oven to 350°F.

In a small mixing bowl, place the graham crackers, margarine, and egg white and mash together with a wooden spoon, until you can form a moist ball. Evenly spread the crust out on the bottom of a 9-inch pie pan.

In the top of a double boiler, place the chocolate and liqueur. Stir the chocolate until completely melted. Set aside but keep warm.

In a blender, place all of the cheesecake ingredients and melted chocolate and mix for 10 to 15 seconds, until creamy. Stop the blender at least once to scrape the sides. Pour the mixture into the pie crust and spread out evenly. Sprinkle the nuts over the top, if desired. Bake for about 1 hour on the middle rack.

Cool to room temperature and refrigerate for 1 to 2 hours before serving.

Makes 8 servings

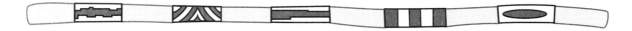

BANANA-RUM RICE PUDDING

Rice pudding is another dessert with a traditionally high-fat, high-calorie history. For this lighter, fruitier version, I replace the heavy cream and eggs with a couple of mashed bananas, a splash of rum, and milk. Banana lovers will adore this treat.

> *3 cups cooked short-grain rice*
> *2 cups milk*
> *¼ cup sugar*
> *½ cup dark raisins or currants*
> *¼ cup dark rum*
> *2 medium bananas, peeled and mashed*
> *½ teaspoon nutmeg*
> *2 to 3 tablespoons pistachio nuts (optional)*

In a large saucepan, combine all of the ingredients (except the nutmeg and nuts) and cook for 15 to 20 minutes over low heat, stirring frequently. Transfer the pudding to a bowl and chill for at least 1 hour before serving.

When you are ready to serve, spoon the rice pudding into bowls and sprinkle with nutmeg. Top with pistachio nuts, if desired.

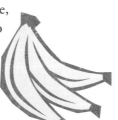

Makes 6 servings

MANGO EGGNOG

Have you ever looked at the ingredients in the typical eggnog? Cream, sugar, and raw eggs. It screams out *cholesterol*. I invented this fruity alternative for a guest appearance I made on "Alive and Wellness," a nationwide cable television show devoted to healthful lifestyles. It was a big hit.

> *1 ripe mango, peeled, pitted, and chopped*
> *1 to 2 medium bananas, peeled and chopped*
> *2 cups chilled rice milk or vanilla soy milk*
> *2 to 3 tablespoons dark rum*
> *1 tablespoon honey*
> *1 teaspoon vanilla extract*
> *½ teaspoon nutmeg*

In a blender, combine all of the ingredients and mix for about 15 seconds, until creamy. Pour into glasses and serve at once.

Makes 4 servings

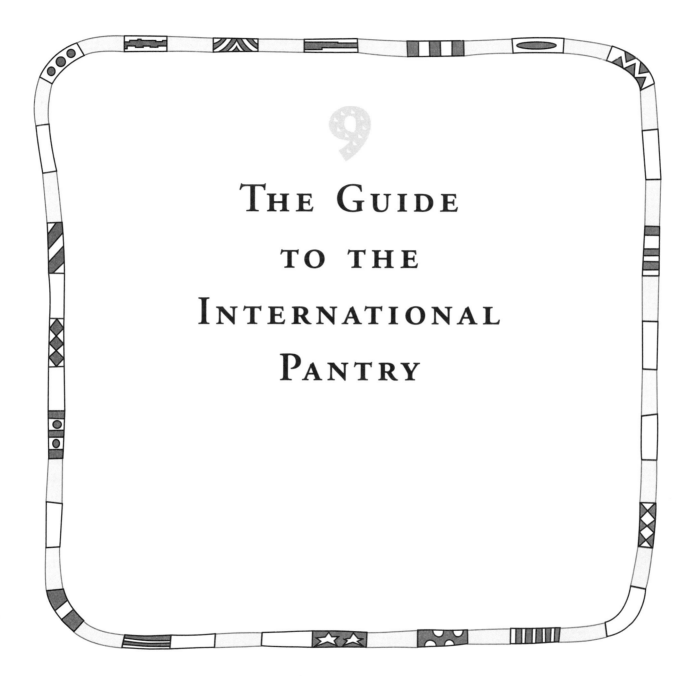

9

THE GUIDE
TO THE
INTERNATIONAL
PANTRY

Here are some valuable ingredients that reside in the well-stocked kitchen and pantry. Some are year-round staples, while others are season-oriented.

GARDEN HERBS

Fresh herbs are the flowers of the spice world; they leave an aromatic scent in the kitchen and a perfumelike residue on your hands, not to mention the vitalizing role they play in the meal. Herbs can amplify flavors in ways that table salt and butter never dreamed possible.

ARUGULA. Also known as rocket or roquette, this long, narrow leaf has a peppery personality that is more pronounced in its larger leaves. It spruces up tossed salads, cold pasta, braised greens, and soups. Arugula can replace basil or cilantro in some dishes.

BASIL. This herb possesses a sharp, cleansing scent with underlying hints of licorice, anise, and mint. The versatile herb is best known for use in pesto, but can jazz up tomato-based soups and sauces, bean salads, stir-fries, and grain dishes. Thai basil and opal (purple) basil are appealing varieties.

CILANTRO. It looks like parsley, but the resemblance ends there. The herb delivers a sharp, pungent, palate-cleansing flavor. It is a favorite spice in Indian, Mexican, Caribbean, and African cooking. Use it in salsas, guacamoles, soups, curries, and bean salads. Cilantro is also known as Chinese parsley and coriander.

EPAZOTE. This narrow leaf has mild hints of mint, oregano, and cilantro. It is primarily used in Mexican bean dishes; it is said to reduce gastric distress.

MARJORAM. This herb is often confused with oregano. It has a sweet, resinlike flavor and is interchangeable with oregano.

MINT. This refers to a family of herbs, all with refreshing, eternally springlike scents: apple, pineapple, orange, spearmint, and peppermint are some of the varieties. It's great in yogurt dips, salads, bean and grain dishes, desserts, and beverages, or for munching on after a meal.

OREGANO. This tiny, oval-shaped herb has a subtle, resinlike flavor. It's more commonly used dried, but fresh oregano offers interesting dynamics. It's similar to marjoram in flavor and appearance.

PARSLEY. Here's an herb that needs no introduction. Originally chewed after a meal as a breath freshener, this omnipresent herb has a myriad of uses and brightens almost any dish.

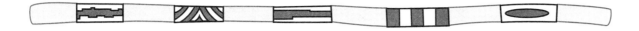

There are two varieties: the common curly leaf and the slightly stronger-flavored flat leaf.

ROSEMARY. This herb has a needlelike shape and a bucolic quality. It exudes a strong pine tree fragrance. Rosemary perks up roasted potatoes, Jerusalem artichokes, carrots, and roasted vegetables.

THYME. The tiny oval petals of this herb have an earthy, pungent scent with rustic undertones. It's one of the few herbs to retain most of its flavor during the cooking process. Common thyme is the most popular, but there is also lemon thyme, pineapple thyme, and others. It's great for soups, stews, marinades, vinaigrettes, and roasted vegetables.

WATERCRESS. This delicate round leaf adds a tangy taste of spring to leafy green salads, dressings, tabouleh, salsas, and soups.

CHILI PEPPERS

Chili peppers enliven, enhance, and in general, turn up the volume of a dish. Connoisseurs of chilies attest to their life-affirming properties and their searing, penetrating, and exhilarating effects on food and on the human condition.

Chilies are high in Vitamins A and C and in other nutrients. Chilies are also low in fat and sodium, and their intense flavor reduces the need for salt or butter. Look for chilies that have smooth, taut skins and are free of blemishes or wrinkles.

To prepare a chili, remove the stem and slit the pepper in half lengthwise. Slide a butter knife along the inside of the pepper, removing the seeds. The pepper is now ready to be minced or chopped. If you have sensitive skin, it is a good idea to wear plastic or rubber gloves when handling the peppers.

If a chili makes your meal too hot, the best remedy is to drink or eat a dairy product such as milk or yogurt. Dairy products have a protein, casein, that washes away capsaicin, the element that produces the chili's heat. Here are samplings of popular chilies.

ANAHEIM. Grown in California, this is a mild, pale green variety of the New Mexico chili. It is an ideal choice for stuffing and other mild dishes.

CAYENNE. This long, slender red chili has a sharp piquant flavor. It is a favorite pod in Creole, African, and Asian cuisines. Cayenne is often dried and ground into powder.

CHIPOTLE. The chipotle is actually a large jalapeño pepper that has been dried and smoked. It's available canned and ready to use or dried and air packed (soak the air-packed chili for at least 30 minutes in warm water before using). This chili offers a concentrated smoky heat and is a good substitute for bacon, pork, or dried meats.

HABANERO. Be careful. This notorious chili is considered to be the world's hottest pod. It is curvaceous, bright, and lantern-shaped and delivers a burning, screeching heat and floral flavor. It is most often orange, but can also be green, red, or yellow. Habaneros are prevalent in Caribbean, Yucatan, and South American cooking. Use them judiciously in marinades, soups, salsas, and sauces.

JALAPEÑO. This dark green, thick-skinned, bullet-shaped chili has a vegetablelike flavor and moderate heat. It is one of the most versatile and widely available chilies, and is good for spicing up everything from salsas, soups, and salads to sauces, pastas, and grain dishes.

NEW MEXICO. This long, tapered green or red chili is native to the American Southwest. The chili produces a symphonic heat and fruity flavor; some argue that there is no equal. It is frequently roasted and stuffed or added to sauces, soups, and rice and bean dishes. When dried, these chilies are tied into a ristra, forming a holiday wreath.

PEPPERONCINI. This pickled, pale green Italian pepper is often found on salad bars. It has a fleeting heat and is great for pasta salads, bean dishes, and grain salads.

POBLANO. This large, forest green and purple pod is shaped like an anvil and has a thick flesh. It has a raisinlike flavor and a mellow heat that sneaks up on you. Poblanos are often roasted and stuffed or added to grain and legume dishes. Dried poblanos are called anchos.

RED FRESNO. Similar to a red jalapeño, only slightly hotter, this chili has broader shoulders and tapers to a point. It is excellent for salsas, rice dishes, curries, sauces, dips, and marinades.

SCOTCH BONNET. Also up for title of the world's hottest, this chili, native to Jamaica, is interchangeable with the habanero, and is just as explosive. Its shape is more contorted than habanero's, and chili aficionados swoon at the sight of them. Use with caution.

SERRANO. This narrow, thin, pointy pepper has a piercing heat that fades quickly but leaves its mark. It is popular in Mexican food, especially salsas, and is almost as prevalent as the jalapeño.

GRAINS AND PASTAS

Grains and pastas form the foundry of meatless cuisine. They contribute bulk, body, nutrients, and amenable flavors to a wide variety of meals from all over the world.

ARBORIO. This short-grained Italian rice is the primary ingredient in risotto, a creamy rice dish. Medium- or short-grained arborio cooks up to a soft, creamy consistency that is perfect for soups and rice pudding. It is available in well-stocked grocery stores, natural food stores, and Italian markets.

BARLEY. This kernel-shaped, mild-flavored grain takes about 40 minutes to cook. Often sold in the pearled form (hulled), it can be cooked like rice and added to soups and hearty entrees.

BASMATI. This is an aromatic, nut-scented, long-grain rice that is prevalent in Indian foods. The rice is fluffy when properly cooked, and it makes a great side dish for curries and other spicy entrees.

BROWN RICE. This rice has its bran still intact. Brown rice has a nutty flavor, a chewy texture, and more fiber and nutrients than polished white rice. It takes 35 to 40 minutes to cook and should be left in the covered pot to steam unheated for another 15 minutes or so.

BULGUR. This popular Middle Eastern grain achieved fame as the basis for tabouleh. Bulgur is made of wheat berries that are precooked, dried, and cracked (it is also called cracked wheat). It's great in legume dishes, light salads, and side dishes and is available in coarse, medium, and fine textures in natural food stores and well-stocked grocery stores.

COUSCOUS. This fabled tiny grain from North Africa is made of fine semolina, a wheat flour used in pasta. It's a boon to the harried cook: the grains take only 10 minutes to cook in hot water. Couscous makes a light staple for salads and side dishes and an appetizing bed for main dishes.

JASMINE RICE. This is an intensely fragrant, nutty white rice with a popcornlike aroma. The grain is similar to basmati, only stickier. Jasmine is popular in Thai and Indonesian cooking and is an excellent side dish or bed for main courses.

QUINOA. This ancient grain is native to the highlands of South America. Quinoa is tiny and ringlike with a nutty flavor, and it expands by volumes when cooked. Quinoa is the closest thing in the grain world to a perfect protein. Like white rice, it cooks up in about 15 minutes. Rinse quinoa thoroughly to wash away the

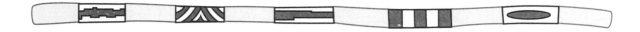

natural but bitter-tasting resin that coats the grains. Pronounced "keen-wa," it is great for salads, main entrees, and side dishes, and it's available in natural food stores and well-stocked grocery stores.

RICE NOODLES. This is a quick-cooking pasta used in Asian meals. It's available as thin noodles (called rice sticks or vermicelli) and as flat, fettucinilike noodles. Rice noodles are sold in Asian markets and well-stocked supermarkets.

SOBA. These long, thin, flat Japanese noodles resemble spaghetti. They are usually made from buckwheat flour, and they're sometimes called buckwheat noodles. They are ideal for soups and salads.

SOMEN. These thin, quick-cooking white Japanese noodles resemble capellini. They are often used for cold salads.

UDON. These Japanese noodles have a long, flat appearance that is similar to linguini. They are made from wheat or rice flour. Udon adds body to salads and soups.

WILD RICE. Not really a rice, but the dark seed of the Native American aquatic grass, wild rice is firm and chewy with an extremely nutty flavor, and takes about an hour to cook. Wild rice

should be combined with other grains to temper its strong, earthy flavor.

BEANS, PEAS, AND LENTILS

There is a copious variety of legumes on the market today. Beans, peas, and lentils—members of the legume family—are nutritional powerhouses, packed with fiber, protein, complex carbohydrates, and loads of other good stuff. Legumes are as versatile as vegetables and add substance, texture, and flavor to a variety of meatless meals.

Before cooking, dried beans must be soaked in plenty of water for at least 4 hours (preferably overnight). Always drain the soaked beans and cook them in fresh water. Most beans take about an hour to become tender; lentils take about 45 minutes. Avoid adding salt or acidic ingredients to the beans during the cooking process, as they inhibit the beans' tenderization and water absorption.

About 1½ cups of cooked beans can replace one 15-ounce can of beans called for in recipes throughout this book. Look for reduced-sodium canned beans that have no added sugar. For an in-depth treatment of legumes, I highly recommend *Lean Bean Cuisine*, the definitive guide to cooking with legumes.

ANASAZI BEANS. These slightly kidney-shaped beans have a reddish, purple skin and mottled, creamy white streaks. These ancient beans were grown by Anasazi Indians in Colorado and in the American Southwest, and are still sold at farmers' markets there today.

BLACK BEANS. Medium-sized and oval-shaped, with an earthy, woodsy flavor, these multipurpose beans are prevalent in Latin America, the Caribbean, Brazil, Mexico, and South and Central America. They are one of my favorites.

BLACK-EYED PEAS. This medium-size, roundish bean has a creamy coffee color and a dark "eye" on its ridge. Savory, earthy, and smooth-flavored, these beans are used in the foods of the American South, Africa, the Caribbean, India, and Middle East.

CHICKPEAS. Also called garbanzo beans and ceci beans, these tan, cream-colored beans have a chewy texture and a nutty taste. They are common in Mediterranean, Indian, Caribbean, and Middle Eastern dishes.

CRANBERRY BEANS. Also called Roman beans, they are medium-size beans with a speckled, cranberry-colored skin that turns solid pink when cooked. Similar to pinto beans in flavor,

they are common in Italian, South American, and Native American cooking.

LENTILS. These beans might be best known for inspiring dal, a curried Indian dish. There are all kinds of lentils—brown, green, red, yellow, and so on. Lentils have a narrow oval shape similar to a thin disc. They are used in Indian, Middle Eastern, North African, and European cooking.

PIGEON PEAS. Also called gungo peas and *gandules*, these small, roundish, brownish-yellow beans have tiny eyes and faint freckles. They are a favorite Caribbean staple.

RED KIDNEY BEANS. Also called Mexican beans, this bean takes its name from its kidneylike shape. Rich and full-flavored with either dark or light red hues, it is enjoyed throughout Latin America, the Caribbean, and Creole countries.

WHITE BEANS. This group of beans includes Great Northern, white kidney beans (cannellini beans), and small oval Navy Beans. Favored in European kitchens, these are popular in casseroles, notably Boston baked beans.

LEAFY GREEN VEGETABLES

Leafy green vegetables offer a mother lode of nutrients and flavor. As this book attests, there

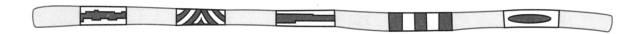

is a large galaxy of leafy greens, and their uses extend well beyond salads to include everything from soups, stews, and grain dishes to braised side dishes.

BOK CHOY. This is a Chinese green with floppy leaves, a wide, white stem, and a subtle cabbage flavor. *Tat soi* is a similar green with smaller leaves.

CHARD. This red or green leaf is often referred to as Swiss chard. It has a crunchy texture; the red chard has beet-red veins throughout the leaf. It can be cooked or eaten raw.

CURLY ENDIVE. Also called chicory, this green has a crunchy, slightly bitter taste. It is best mixed with other greens.

ESCAROLE. A wide leaf lettuce with a mild flavor used in Italian cuisine, this most versatile leafy green is good for soups and pasta sauces.

FRISEE. Also called French chicory, this is a delicate, mildly flavored green worth trying in a mesclun salad.

KALE. This underrated olive green leaf is often used as a garnish. Try it in soups, sauces, and rice dishes. Although it may be eaten raw, it tastes better when cooked.

MESCLUN. This is the French term for "mixed field greens." It is typically a mixture of young tender leaves of radicchio, lamb's ear, endive, chard, red and green leaf lettuces, frisee, mizuna, and other exotic and basic greens.

MIZUNA. This is a narrow, fernlike Japanese mustard green with a flavor similar to arugula and frisee. It can be cooked or eaten raw.

PURSLANE. Some people think of this as a weed because of its rampant growth tendencies. The tender leaves have a delicate flavor and are rich in many vitamins. Mix it in with a salad of other mixed greens or mesclun.

SOUTHERN GREENS. (Mustard, collard, turnip, dandelion, and beet greens.) These versatile greens have varying degrees of mustardlike flavors and a slight bitterness. Most cook up quickly (collards take 20 to 30 minutes) and can be added to one-pot meals, soups, and stews, or can be braised by themselves.

WINTER SQUASH AND ROOT VEGETABLES

There are a bounty of winter squash and root vegetables that inspire wonderful soups, stews, casseroles, sweet quick breads, and mashed and

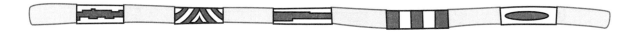

roasted dishes. Winter squash are rich in beta-carotene and other nutrients; root vegetables are valuable sources of complex carbohydrates. Although most have long shelf lives, it is still important to choose specimens that are blemish free and firm, with taut, unbroken skins.

ACORN. This aptly-named, attractive squash is shaped like an acorn. Its dark skin is sometimes flecked with golden streaks. The orange flesh has a mild, smooth flavor.

BEET ROOTS. These magenta orbs have the versatility of a potato and the crisp flavor of a green vegetable. Look for beets with their green tops still attached—the beet greens are an added bonus. Beets can be shredded raw and tossed into a salad or roasted whole. They are best known for their role in borscht, the Russian bisque.

BUTTERCUP. A dark, green-skinned gourd with a squatty, turban-shape, this has a sweet, buttery flesh and is interchangeable with most squash.

LEEKS. Looking like the large, clumsy offspring of an onion and a scallion, leeks have a mild oniony flavor. They should be thoroughly soaked and rinsed before cooking to remove any gritty sand caught between the coarse leaves.

BUTTERNUT. This is the most common squash. It is long, narrow, and tan-skinned with a bell-shaped end. It is widely available, versatile, and tasty.

PARSNIPS. This root looks like an albino carrot. Parsnips have a mild, slightly sweet, starchy flavor and a firm, crunchy texture. Try using it in place of a potato.

PUMPKIN. The small sugar pie varieties of pumpkin have a dense, rich flesh; the larger field pumpkins ("jack-o'-lanterns") are mildly flavored and more seedy. (Sugar pie pumpkins are most commonly used for cooking, but I use both varieties.)

RED KURI. This large, orangish-red squash has a thin skin and a delectable, dense flesh. Its flavor and density are similar to a Hubbard squash or a West Indian pumpkin. This squash is also known as Golden Hubbard.

RUTABAGA. This large, softball-sized, earth-toned orb has a firm, yellowish flesh with a mild cauliflower flavor. The bulbous root is often covered with a thin coat of wax (paraffin) to extend its shelf life—the wax should be peeled off before cooking.

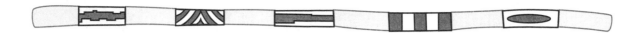

SUGAR LOAF, SWEET DUMPLING, AND DELI-CATA. These small, sweet, buttery-tasting squash are good for single-portion servings. Roasting is the most common method of cooking them.

TURNIPS. These roundish, off-white orbs have a light purple band around the top. They have a firm texture and a subtle radish flavor. The greens are edible as well.

WEST INDIAN PUMPKIN. This large, Hubbard-like squash has vibrant orange flesh and a sweet potatolike flavor. It is often sold in wedges in Caribbean and Hispanic markets and in well-stocked supermarkets. It is also called calabaza.

EXOTIC FRUITS AND VEGETABLES

In recent years the produce aisles of grocery stores have exploded with all kinds of fascinating fruits and vegetables. This is great news for cooks in search of high adventure in the kitchen.

CHAYOTE. This pale green, pear-shaped, gnarly squash is prevalent in Caribbean and Creole cooking. It can replace summer squash in soups and sauté dishes; it also makes for an extremely moist sweet bread. Chayote is also known as cho cho, christophene, and mirliton.

DASHEEN. This tuber is similar to a potato. It has a barklike skin and a white flesh with light purple specks. Also called taro, dasheen is used in soups, stews, and chip dips.

GINGERROOT. A gnarly root with clean, sharp, perfumelike essence, it is widely used in African, Asian, Caribbean, and Indian food. Gingerroot should be chopped fine before adding to curries, stir-fries, soups, and salads. Dried gingerroot is a pale substitute.

JICAMA. Also called a Mexican potato, this brown-skinned tuber has an extremely moist, crisp white flesh with a mild, water chestnut flavor. It is perfect for shredding and adding to salads and coleslaw. It is best eaten raw.

MANGOES. This is the quintessential tropical fruit. A ripe mango invokes the flavors of pineapple, citrus, and nectarine. It is kidney-shaped with a green skin marked with reddish-orange spots and a coral, beta-carotene rich flesh. Like an avocado, a ripe mango should give a little when pressed. Green, unripe mangoes are crunchy and not as sweet.

PAPAYA. This light green and coral-hued fruit has a flesh similar to cantaloupe. It contains a

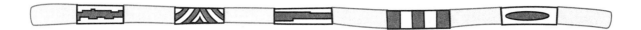

natural enzyme, papain, which aids in digestion. Papaya adds a fruity tropical nuance to salads, cold sauces, and dressings. To eat, scoop out the inner black seeds and peel off the thin skin.

PLANTAINS. These large, motley, thick-skinned members of the banana family are a prominent starch in the Caribbean and Africa. Plantains must be cooked to be eaten. Green plantains, not yet ripe, resemble a starchy, chalky potato and are used in soups; ripe, yellow plantains are sweet and bananalike and are quite desirable when roasted.

STAR FRUIT. This sweet-and-tart, thirst-quenching tropical fruit is star-shaped when cut widthwise, hence the name. Also called carambola, this fruit can be added to fruit salads and green salads or eaten out of hand. It ripens from tart green to citrusy sweet when yellow.

TOMATILLOS. Also called Mexican tomatoes, tomatillos are similar to green tomatoes in flavor and appearance, with more of a sour flavor. Peel off the paperlike husk and add the fruit to salsas and sauces.

YUCA. This sturdy, brown-skinned, white-fleshed root is often coated with a protective layer of wax. Also called cassava, yuca adds a starchy sustenance to many Caribbean soups and stews. Processed yuca forms the basis of tapioca.

THE WELL-STOCKED SHELF

BALSAMIC VINEGAR. A premium, well-aged vinegar with a smooth, balanced, low acidic taste, balsamic vinegar endows a salad with instant class.

CANOLA OIL. This versatile oil has the lowest saturated fat content of vegetable oils and a high Omega-3 content. Also known as rapeseed oil, it is widely used for cooking and baking and in dressings and marinades.

KETJAP MANIS. This sweetened, syrupy version of soy sauce is prominent in Indonesian cooking. Pour it over rice, bean, and potato dishes. You can blend 1 teaspoon of brown sugar or molasses with 1 tablespoon light soy sauce for an approximate substitute. Look for ketjap manis in Asian grocery stores.

MISO. A thick paste of fermented soybeans, salt, and grains, miso is used to flavor Japanese soups, sauces, and dressings. It is rich in protein and has a mild flavor. Miso is said to facilitate digestion. The most common varieties are barley (red), rice (white), and soy (dark). Miso is available in natural food stores and Asian markets.

OLIVE OIL. This premium oil has a strong, musky olive flavor. It contains monounsaturated fat, which is good news for people on reduced cholesterol diets. Extra virgin olive oil comes from the first pressing of olives and is cherished for its refined fruity presence. Use it sparingly as a salad dressing or as a dip for bread. The next level, pure olive oil, is typically used for cooking and dressings.

RED WINE VINEGAR. This workhorse of vinegars is used in vinaigrettes, chutneys, marinades, and salads of all kinds. Almost any brand will do for most recipes.

RICE VINEGAR. This mild, smoothly flavored clear vinegar is prominently used in Asian dishes and in salads.

SAMBAL. This is an Indonesian chili paste with an addictive "sweet heat" style of flavor. Serve it with rice dishes and as a spicy topping for soups and stews. It is sold in many Asian grocery stores.

SCOTCH BONNET PEPPER SAUCE OR HABANERO SAUCE. This is a fiery hot liquid with an enormous potential to fry your taste buds; if overdone, it could obliterate the meal. When used properly, it is an elixir of bliss to connoisseurs of hot food. Avoid it if you prefer bland or mild fare.

SEITAN. This is a wheat product without the starch, which leaves the gluten. It is referred to as a meat substitute because of its protein density and chewiness. It is most often used in sandwiches, soups, stews, and curries. Look for it in the refrigerated sections of well-stocked grocery stores and natural food stores.

SOY SAUCE. This is a dark, salty, and distinctly flavored liquid used in a variety of Asian sauces, soups, stir-fries, and rice dishes. When shopping, choose a light soy sauce with reduced-sodium content and without any added sugar or MSG.

TABASCO OR OTHER BOTTLED HOT SAUCES. This piquant vinegary liquid is made from the fermented mash of Tabasco peppers (and sometimes other chilies, depending on the brand). It is an antidote for the bland or mundane dishes of the world. To some, it is a replacement for salty or buttery flavors.

TAHINI. A smooth sesame seed paste with the consistency of thick pancake batter. It is a cherished flavor in many Middle Eastern dips and sauces including hummus and baba ghanoush.

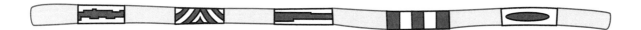

TOFU. A protein-rich soybean curd (it is also called bean curd), tofu has a mild, unobtrusive flavor with textures varying from extra firm to soft (or silken). This versatile ingredient can be used in soups, salads, main entrees, and even cheesecakes. It is usually stored in water and refrigerated.

WINE MUSTARD. More commonly known as Dijon-style mustard, this table condiment thickens and enlivens salad dressings and sauces and is an indispensable ingredient in the basic vinaigrette recipe.

INDEX

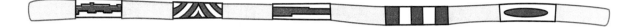

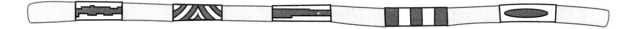

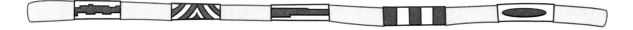

ABOUT THE AUTHOR

Upon graduating from Cornell University in 1983, Jay Solomon opened a successful chocolate chip cookie business. He then opened a gourmet cookie and sandwich shop, followed some years later by Jay's Cafe, a full-service restaurant specializing in healthful tropical cuisine and featuring Caribbean, Latin American, and Pacific Rim fare. He was the chef and owner of Jay's Cafe for seven years before selling it in 1992.

Jay has taught adult cooking classes for several years and leads "Adventures-in-Cooking" seminars in Ithaca, New York. He has also been featured guest chef in schools in Boston, Baltimore, Philadelphia, and cities throughout the East Coast. Jay has appeared regularly on "Alive and Wellness," a cable television show on the America's Talking Network, and other nationwide shows. In addition, his food articles and recipes frequently appear in *Vegetarian Times*, *Restaurants USA*, and other national magazines. This is his fifth cookbook.